Advanced Practice in Nursing

Under the Auspices of the *International Council of Nurses (ICN)*

Series Editor:
Christophe Debout
GIP-IFITS
Health Chair Sciences-Po Paris/IDS UMR Inserm 1145
Paris, France

This series of concise monographs, endorsed by the International Council of Nurses, explores various aspects of advanced nursing practice at the international level.

The ICN International Nurse Practitioner/Advanced Practice Nursing Network definition has been adopted for this series to define advanced nursing practice: "A Nurse Practitioner/Advanced Practice Nurse is a registered nurse who has acquired the expert knowledge base, complex decision-making skills and clinical competencies for expanded practice, the characteristics of which are shaped by the context and/or country in which s/he is credentialed to practice. A master's degree is recommended for entry level."

At the international level, advanced practice nursing practice encompasses two professional profiles:

Nurse practitioners (NPs) who have mastered advanced nursing practice, and are capable of diagnosing, making prescriptions for and referring patients. Though they mainly work in the community, some also work in hospitals. Clinical nurse specialists (CNSs) are expert nurses who deliver high-quality nursing care to patients and promote quality care and performance in nursing teams.

The duties performed by these two categories of advanced practice nurses on an everyday basis can be divided into five interrelated roles:

Clinical practice

Consultation

Education

Leadership

Research

The series addresses four topics directly related to advanced nursing practice:

APN in practice (NPs and CNSs)

Education and continuous professional development for advanced practice nurses

Managerial issues related to advanced nursing practice

Policy and regulation of advanced nursing practice

The contributing authors are mainly APNs (NPs and CNSs) recruited from the ICN International Nurse Practitioner/Advanced Practice Nursing Network. They include clinicians, educators, researchers, regulators and managers, and are recognized as experts in their respective fields.

Each book within the series reflects the fundamentals of nursing / advanced nursing practice and will promote evidence-based nursing.

More information about this series at http://www.springer.com/series/13871

Laserina O'Connor

The Nature of Scholarship, a Career Legacy Map and Advanced Practice

An Important Triad

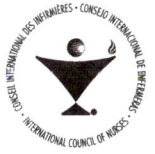

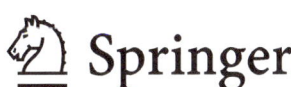

Laserina O'Connor
UCD School of Nursing
Midwifery and Health Systems
University College Dublin (UCD)
Belfield
Dublin
Ireland

ISSN 2511-3917   ISSN 2511-3925   (electronic)
Advanced Practice in Nursing
ISBN 978-3-319-91694-1   ISBN 978-3-319-91695-8   (eBook)
https://doi.org/10.1007/978-3-319-91695-8

This Springer imprint is published by the registered company Springer Nature Switzerland AG
The registered company address is: Gewerbestrasse 11, 6330 Cham, Switzerland

Foreword

Recently, I had the privilege of opening the 10th International Council of Nurses (ICN) NP/APN conference held in the Netherlands. Over a thousand advanced practice nurses from all over the world attended this event which focused on nursing's role in transforming care, with particular reference to the sustainable development goals (SDGs) and human resources for health. I could not have been prouder listening to the presentations and stories told by nurses about the work that they were accomplishing in providing better health outcomes to patients and communities.

But there is still so much more to be done. As a commissioner on the Independent High-Level Commission for Non-Communicable Diseases, it is clear that the world will not meet the targets set out in the SDGs of reducing premature death from non-communicable diseases (NCDs) by 30% by 2030 unless the challenge is addressed differently. We need governments, health systems, public and private organisations to mobilise the nursing workforce, to harness its value and to unleash the profession's true potential. Nursing will be pivotal in the fight for better access to quality and affordable care that will improve health outcomes across the world.

Today, the advanced practice nursing workforce is growing at a rapid rate. Whilst this expanse may have started because of the evolution of professionals to meet the increasing service needs and shortfalls in healthcare providers, it is now growing because of the enormous benefits that the profession provides through its approach to health and wellbeing. We know that health systems are at their strongest when they are supported by skilled, educated nurses in sufficient numbers where there are supportive cultures in place.

At times, the profession has been required to adjust to differences in countries' service needs, education and regulation. This has led to some confusion over the exact role and scope of the advanced practice nurse. However, now is the time to capitalise on the research and evidence behind the role of advanced practice nursing.

This book, the third in a series developed by Springer, on the subject of advanced practice nursing is significant to the progression of advanced practice nursing around the world. Authored by Professor Laserina O'Connor, the book is for educators, regulators, advanced practice nurses and those considering or aspiring to move into this distinguished profession.

The Nature of Scholarship, a Career Legacy Map and Advanced Practice provides a compelling and powerful vision of nursing that is supported by scientific reading and academic scholarship. Through the lens of nursing, Professor O'Connor showcases the importance of patient-centred care, its relationship to advanced practice nursing and the connection to nursing scholarship. The relationship between the nurse and the patient and the approach to care and practice is what makes nursing unique amongst the health professions. As nurses, we celebrate this and use this relationship as the foundation for our practice.

The book also importantly sets a challenge to the profession. We know that the complexity of health challenges and issues cannot be solved by yesterday's reasoning. Professor O'Connor, through the exploration of Boyer's work, compels and leads us to think differently. It highlights a vision and roadmap that seeks to increase nursing contribution to the challenges that lay ahead by encouraging education, innovative and creative thinking which can be achieved through scholarship.

I am honoured to endorse this book. Globally relevant, it further progresses the vital role of nursing. I also hope that it aids and inspires future nurses to take on the role of APN and use their skills and talents to create a healthier world.

Annette Kennedy
President International Council of Nurses
Geneva, Switzerland

Foreword

The healthcare systems in many developed countries face enormous challenges in preventing and treating non-communicable, lifestyle-related diseases, treating anti-microbial resistant infections, and meeting the healthcare needs of ageing and under-served populations. These challenges exist in circumstances of ever-increasing healthcare costs that include the costs associated with educating and training health care professionals. A key challenge for most national health systems is securing and retaining suitably qualified healthcare professionals and supporting them to continually develop and maintain their knowledge and skills in providing safe, evidence-informed and effective treatments and the highest standards of care that healthcare consumers demand and expect.

In many countries, nurses have demonstrated their readiness to address these challenges through expanding the scope of their professional practice, thereby assuming greater responsibility, accountability and professional autonomy in their practice. Expanded scope of practice is best exemplified in the movement for advanced practice, a movement that has resulted in a more flexible and responsive professional with greater professional autonomy but capable of engaging in more deliberate and meaningful collaborative practice with physicians and other health professionals. With greater autonomy comes greater responsibility for professional decision making, and as both autonomous and interdisciplinary practitioners, advanced nurse practitioners must not only engage in independent professional decision making but must do so from a standpoint of criticality that is informed by advanced knowledge and insights that, in turn, inform their practice. Such criticality is expressed through scholarship, a synthesis of expert clinical practice; interdisciplinary consultation; practice innovation; research, writing and dissemination; and the use of digital technology and other media to communicate ideas. Scholarship is fundamental to the conduct of advanced nursing practice, whether that practice involves direct nursing interventions or coordinating and directing the work of other practitioners and carers.

Laserina O'Connor's book is a timely and welcome analysis of scholarship and its application in the field of advanced nursing practice. It clearly sets out the nature of scholarship; expands on the various forms of scholarship, as described by Boyer; examines how the forms are interrelated; and analyses how the forms intersect at the point of practice. As a book aimed at individual advanced nurse practitioners and aspirant advanced nurse practitioners, it also offers a roadmap for professional self-development and advancement. When advanced practitioners are clear as to their own intended contribution to healthcare, they hold a professional legacy and they are more likely to create and attain their legacy if they develop a legacy map for self-guidance. This book offers practical guidelines for developing such a map, showing advanced nurse practitioners and aspirant advanced nurse practitioners the steps involved in mapping out their own career outcomes against their career goals and aspirations and their practice capacities.

The book also offers professional regulators a cogent account of and a vision for scholarship and its application in advanced practice; this account should therefore inform regulators in their efforts to define the range of practice competencies and professional attributes for advanced practitioners. In a wider sense, the book represents the kind of scholarly contribution that is sometimes lacking in modern professional discourse, namely a distinctly *nursing* discourse that is epistemically strong. It offers a powerful vision of scientific nursing, and in so doing, it represents a treatise on the confluence of academic and professional nursing that is markedly grounded in the discipline of nursing in its writing.

As a professor of clinical nursing, a registered advanced nurse practitioner in pain management and a registered nurse prescriber, Laserina O'Connor brings a rich professional biography, a repertoire of academic and clinical talents, and a depth of experience in clinical practice, research and teaching to the writing of this important and timely text. As a clinical leader with an international profile in her field of practice, she represents an exemplar of individual contribution and impact, and as an academic practitioner, she demonstrates the essential characteristics of a scholar and teacher. Through her book, she brings these roles together to provide an indispensable lifelong development guide for other advanced practitioners.

O'Connor also articulates a distinct disciplinary perspective on scholarship, which can better inform other health professionals of the distinct nursing contribution to health care, research and practice improvement. In so doing, she contributes to enhanced interdisciplinary understanding and solidarity, essential, if the challenges in healthcare are to be met. Through her own personal reflections as someone who holds a joint academic-clinical appointment, O'Connor offers a context-bound analysis and real-world reflections on what it means to practice at the level of advanced practice. Her book presents scholarship as a real and meaningful process in the conduct of advanced practice, and it clearly establishes the patient as the focus of that practice.

This expertly written book is a major achievement in bringing together a coherent and vibrant synthesis of three distinct but interrelated topics: scholarship, career legacy mapping and advanced practice. It is a vital contribution of international significance, representing, as it does, the current state of development of modern professional nursing. It is an essential book for advanced nurse practitioners, educators and professional regulators.

Professor Gerard M. Fealy, PhD, RGN
Professor of Nursing and Head of School
UCD School of Nursing, Midwifery and Health Systems
University College Dublin
Dublin, Ireland

Acknowledgements

I am deeply indebted to Christophe Debout who invited me to write a book on advanced practice nursing based on my passionate presentation on the topic during an international week for students held in Paris, France. Christophe was the glue that made certain the topic was thought-provoking.

My sincere thanks to David Stewart, whose attention to detail when reading the manuscript afforded me the opportunity to make this book a worthy read for educators, regulators, advanced practice nursing practitioners/aspirants and others who are privileged to be a part of and continue to have an impact on the patient's/client's care trajectory.

Paula Byrne Purcell for her efforts in preparing the visual illustrations, which are a great contribution to the text.

Nathalie LHorset-Poulain at Springer, who has been patient, thoughtful, encouraging and thorough in the preparation and printing of this book.

Special and sincere thanks to Mr Rajesh Gopalakrishnan, the ever-patient program manager and Ms Beauty Christobel Gunasekaran, production editor.

Finian, Cillian and Zoe, I owe my greatest debt.

Finally to John, forever in my heart.

Disclosure

The views and opinions expressed in this book are those of the author and do not necessarily reflect the official policy or position of the ICN.

Contents

1 The Nature of Scholarship 1
  1.1 Introduction 1
  1.2 The Landscape of Scholarship............................... 1
      1.2.1 Characteristics of Scholarship 3
      1.2.2 Research and Scholarship Are Almost Synonymous 5
      1.2.3 The Scholarship of Discovery 5
      1.2.4 The Scholarship of Teaching 6
      1.2.5 Scholarship of Integration 7
      1.2.6 Scholarship of Application........................... 8
      1.2.7 Scholarship of Engagement 9
  1.3 Framing the Scholarship of Engagement Within Communities
     of Practice 9
  1.4 Conclusion 12
  References.. 13

2 Boyer's Pillars of Scholarship 17
  2.1 Introduction 17
  2.2 Context of Boyer's Pillars of Scholarship 17
      2.2.1 The Scholarship of Discovery 18
      2.2.2 Scholarship of Engagement 18
      2.2.3 Scholarship of Teaching............................. 20
      2.2.4 Scholarship of Integration 22
      2.2.5 Scholarship of Application........................... 23
      2.2.6 Scholarship of Practice 24
  2.3 Clinical Scholarship....................................... 25
  2.4 Conclusion 26
  References.. 27

**3 Transforming Advanced Practice Nursing into
Clinical Scholarship** 31
  3.1 Introduction 31
  3.2 Pillars of Scholarship and Clinical Scholarship.............. 31
      3.2.1 Clinical Scholarship Is Elusive in Nursing 33
      3.2.2 Essential Standards to Adjudicate on Scholarly Work...... 35

	3.3	Scholarship of Practice	38
	3.4	Conclusion	41
	References		42

4 **The Spectrum of Clinical Scholarship** 45
    4.1   Introduction 45
    4.2   Clinical Scholarship...................................... 45
          4.2.1   Definitions Surrounding the Milieu of Clinical
                    Scholarship.................................... 47
          4.2.2   Patient Centered Care 51
          4.2.3   Definitions and Dimensions of Patient-Centered Care 53
          4.2.4   Communities of Practice Support A Culture of Clinical
                    Scholarship.................................... 61
    4.3   Conclusion 64
    References... 65

5 **Doctorate of Nursing Practice: A Conduit for Scholarship**
in the Realm of Advanced Practice 71
    5.1   Introduction 71
    5.2   Doctoral and Professional Education for Advanced Practice
          Links to Boyer's Model 71
    5.3   Doctor of Nursing Practice: Scholarship Revisited 73
    5.4   Evolution from First to Second to Third Generation Professional
          Doctorates 77
    5.5   Engaging in the Scholarship of Practice 81
    5.6   Scholarship in Advanced Practice Nursing 85
    5.7   Conclusion 87
    References... 88

6 **Career Legacy Cartography Portfolio for Advanced**
Practice Nursing 93
    6.1   Introduction 93
    6.2   The Science of Cartography................................ 93
    6.3   Career Cartography and the Scholarship Trajectory 94
    6.4   Applying the Science of Cartography to Advanced
          Practice Nursing... 95
    6.5   Career Legacy Portfolio for Advanced Practice Nursing
          Practitioners/Aspirants.................................... 97
    6.6   Professional Profile: Statement of Responsibilities.............. 98
    6.7   The Creativity (Creative) Contract........................... 99
    6.8   Professional Profile: Biographical Sketch 99
    6.9   Components of Career Cartography 100
          6.9.1   Destination Statement/Legacy 100
          6.9.2   Identification of the Policy Context..................... 101
          6.9.3   Career Legacy Map 102
          6.9.4   Goals 103

6.9.5   Concept Mapping.   103
6.9.6   Placing the Legacy/Destination Statement   105
6.9.7   Career Cartography: Mapping Variations   106
6.9.8   Establishing a Supportive Career Legacy
         Cartography Team   106
6.9.9   Communicating and Disseminating Science   108
6.10   Professional Profile: Selected Samples of Scholarly Work   108
         6.10.1 Challenges in the Legacy Mapping Process   109
6.11   Career Legacy Portfolio Toolkit.   111
         6.11.1 Professional Profile: Statement of Responsibilities.   111
         6.11.2 Professional Profile: Biographical Sketch   112
         6.11.3 Professional Profile: Selected Samples of Scholarly
                 Work.   129
         6.11.4 Professional Profile: Biographical Profile Continued
                 Capabilities and Competences.   131
         6.11.5 Advanced Practice Nursing Practitioner Schema
                 of Metrics and Associated Indicators.   134
6.12   Conclusion   135
References/Bibliography.   136
   Appendices of Portfolio   136
References.   136

7   **Reflections of a 'Joint Clinical Chair-Advanced Practice
     Nursing Practitioner' on Finding Meaning in a Patient's Story
     Allied with Clinical Scholarship**   139
     7.1   Introduction   139
            7.1.1   Exemplar Case and Context.   139
            7.1.2   Exemplar Case and the Role of the Advanced Practice
                     Nursing Practitioner.   141
     7.2   Reflection Through the Lens of a 'Joint Clinical-Chair-Advanced
            Practice Nursing Practitioner'   142
     7.3   Conclusion   148
     References.   149

Introduction

The dimensions of scholarship outlined by Boyer act as a triangular frame that provides a stable architecture for the nature of scholarship, a career legacy map and advanced practice that weave interdependently throughout this book.

Chapter 1 focuses on the landscape of scholarship and Boyer's vision of tomorrow's scholars who must be liberally educated, think creatively, communicate effectively and have the capacity and the inclination to place ideas in a larger context. Further, the challenges of the various dimensions of Boyer's scholarship are set out in the context of the advanced practice nursing practitioner who is urged not to pay lip service to the scholarship of engagement. Chapter 2 expands on Boyer's pillars of scholarship, and guiding questions are presented in the context of scientific inquiry within discipline-specific silos for reflective consideration by the advanced practice nursing practitioner/aspirant.

Chapter 3 views transforming advanced practice nursing into clinical scholarship using Boyer's pillars as a lever to advance nursing knowledge, and through this advancement of knowledge, patient outcomes become visible. Parallels are drawn between clinical scholarship and the scholarship of application and practice. The qualities of the clinical scholar/practitioner such as integrity, perseverance and courage serve as a reminder that scholarship has a moral aspect in the clinical setting. The essential standards to adjudicate scholarly work are presented as a common arc of intellectual endeavour linked with Boyer's work on evaluating the scholarly activities of the scholar/practitioner.

Chapter 4 focuses on clinical scholarship and diagrammatically represents how the advanced practice nursing practitioner can earn the rites-to-passage towards becoming a scholar practitioner. Patient-centred care is detailed in light of the role of the advanced practice nursing practitioner that necessitates an enabling culture within the healthcare arena and the academy. Further, communities of practice aligned with the scholarship of engagement may well raise the profile of patient-centred care and embrace the deeper meaning of patient-centredness rather than a portion of the term 'patient-centred care'. Chapter 5 centres on the debate surrounding the doctor of nursing practice as an alternative to the doctor of philosophy in the realm of advanced practice nursing. The distinction between researching professionals and professional researchers is presented with a note of caution from the literature that nurse scientists are also relevant to expand the knowledge base of the discipline of nursing. The evolution of various modes of knowledge production doctorates is addressed that also highlights the paucity of empirical literature on such doctorates. Suggestions are presented on the readiness of the clinical milieu for specific outcome measures that are required to capture the advanced practice nursing practitioners' metrics and performance indicators.

Chapter 6 details the science of cartography and its relationship to career cartography. The components of career legacy cartography are presented as they embed in a portfolio. The career legacy mapping process for advanced practice nursing practitioner/aspirant is discussed in-depth, pertinent to five dimensions of scholarship: discovery, integration, engagement, application and teaching. The practicalities of creating a portfolio step-by-step illustrated in a toolkit are provided. Working through the career legacy cartography process in this book will allow the advanced practice nursing practitioner/aspirant push past the boundaries of individual local health outcomes and think about how their work will impact globally.

An exemplar case in clinical practice is explored by a joint-chair of clinical nursing. The complexity of the pain case is unravelled utilising a patient-centred framework. The meaning of the patient story is narrated through the lens of the clinical professor who is also an advanced practice nursing practitioner in pain medicine. The capabilities expected of a clinical professor in practice are put to the test as the case unfolds. The outcome hopefully will provoke conversation among advanced practice nursing practitioners and aspirants on the enablers that nurses bring to the bedside in the context of 'what matters most to the patient as an individual' is 'what matters most to the nurse'. This final chapter is part of the architecture that connects the nature of clinical scholarship, and an advanced practice nursing ethic of inquiry perspective within the pillars of Boyer's dimensions of scholarship.

The Nature of Scholarship

1.1 Introduction

The landscape of scholarship is addressed and the various terms interrelated with scholarship are described in detail. Characteristics of the five dimensions of scholarship are discussed and clinical scholarship is linked within the chapter. A dialogue is presented on the notion that research and scholarship are almost synonymous. Framing the scholarship of engagement with communities of inquiry is explored with particular reference to the acknowledgement of a 'mosaic of talent' in the context of the scholar/practitioner. Further, engaged scholarship implies a fundamental shift in how advanced practice nursing practitioners define their relationship with communities of practice and the methodologies utilised in the production of credible scholarship for the enhanced public good and academic—research—and learning outcomes.

1.2 The Landscape of Scholarship

In *Scholarship Reconsidered, Priorities of the Professoriate*, the proposal put forward was that colleges and universities need a fresher, more capacious vision of scholarship. Boyer (1990) desired that the practice of scholarship be a focus of national discussion, reaching well beyond the ivory tower. He lamented the "publish-or-perish" reality faculty members faced and challenged the nation to reconsider the definition of scholarship. Tomorrow's scholars must be liberally educated, think creatively, communicate effectively, and have the capacity and the inclination to place ideas in a larger context (Boyer 1990, p. 65). Beyond the scholarship of discovering knowledge and integrating knowledge, a third priority was conveyed, the scholarship of sharing knowledge. According to Boyer (1996) scholarship is a communal act, you never get tenured for research alone, you get tenured for research and publication, which means you have to teach somebody what you have learned.

© Springer Nature Switzerland AG 2019
L. O'Connor, *The Nature of Scholarship, a Career Legacy Map and Advanced Practice*, Advanced Practice in Nursing, https://doi.org/10.1007/978-3-319-91695-8_1

Furthermore, academics must continue to communicate not only with their peers but also with future scholars in the classroom in order to keep the flame of scholarship alive (Boyer 1990, p. 16). Colleges/universities according to Glassick et al. (1997) should broaden the scope of scholarship, and set out a new paradigm that views scholarship as having four separate but over-lapping dimensions: the scholarship of discovery, the scholarship of integration, the scholarship of application, and the scholarship of teaching (p. 9).

The first and most familiar element in Boyer's model is the scholarship of discovery and comes closest to what academics mean when they speak of research, although this type of scholarship also embraces the creative work of faculty in the literary, visual, and performing arts (Glassick et al. 1997). Integration, the second of the four forms of scholarship involves faculty making connections within and between disciplines, modifying the contexts in which people view knowledge and offsetting the inclination to split knowledge into ever more cryptic bits and pieces. The scholarship of integration is serious, disciplined work that seeks to interpret, draw together, and bring new insight to bear on original research (Glassick et al. 1997). The third element, the scholarship of application, moves toward engagement as the scholar asks, "How can knowledge be responsibly applied to consequential problems?" (Glassick et al. 1997, p. 9). Theory and practice interact in such ventures and improve each other. Kielhofner (2005a, b) notes that researchers have traditionally expected knowledge created to guide practice. Further, he states "… we have bestowed upon our theory and research the authority to specify what should go in practice while mostly leaving the problem of how to actualize those specifications to the practitioner" (Kielhofner 2005b, p. 232). Finally, the scholarship of teaching initiates students into the best values of the academy, enabling them to understand and contribute more fully in the larger culture (Glassick et al. 1997). In *Scholarship Reconsidered, Priorities of the Professoriate*, there is a proposal that colleges and universities help faculty build on their strengths and sustain their energies by affording them flexible career pathways that avoid narrow definitions of scholarship (Glassick et al. 1997). Whatever the scholarly emphasis, the approach deserves dignity and respect, insofar as it is performed with distinction. Excellence must be the only yardstick (Glassick et al. 1997).

The Canadian Association of Schools of Nursing, (CASN) (2013) position statement on scholarship, defines scholarship as the creation, affirmation, amalgamation, and/or implementation of knowledge intended to advance the discipline of nursing. Specifically, discovery as inquiry leading to new knowledge (original research that advances knowledge); teaching as pedagogical inquiry (discovery, integration, and application); application as discipline-specific knowledge expertise guiding professional practice (using new and synthesised knowledge in problem solving); and integration as the synthesis of knowledge. Furthermore, scholarship involves critical reflection, discipline-specific knowledge expertise and original approaches to themes of interest under study (CASN 2013; Glassick et al. 1997). These position statements expand on Boyer's traditional definition of scholarship that included discovery, teaching, application, and integration.

New challenges-loom large on the horizon, as we move toward a new century (Boyer 1990). Boyer set forth a view of scholarship that he believed was more appropriate to these new looming challenges. "We strongly affirm the importance of research-what we have called the scholarship of discovery. Without the vigorous pursuit of free and open inquiry each country simply will not have the intellectual capacity it needs to resolve the huge, almost intractable social, economic, and ecological problems, both national and global. Nor will the academy itself remain vital if it fails to enlarge its own store of knowledge. But to define the work of the professoriate narrowly-chiefly in terms of the research model-is to deny powerful realities" (Boyer 1990, p. 75). Therefore, 'other forms of scholarship-teaching, integration, and application-must be fully acknowledged and positioned on a more equal footing with discovery. Instead of describing faculty roles in terms of the familiar trilogy of teaching, research and service, the argument was put forward that faculty were responsible for four basic tasks; discovering, integrating, applying and representing the knowledge of their scholarly fields' (Edgerton 2005, xii).

1.2.1 Characteristics of Scholarship

The characteristics of scholarship is associated with high standards of excellence, scientific rigour, and integrity (Newland and Truglio-Londrigan 2003). Scholarship is, in a way, 'an invitation'—a challenge—to reconsider our identity as language educators: it suggests an identity that expands into areas often occluded in the past to one that is more visible, more vocal, making contributions to professional knowledge, exerting influence, shaping practices and policies, engaging with students differently and accumulating social and epistemic capital and recognition (Ding 2016, p. 13). Moreover, Boyer (1990) pointed to the richness of the term 'scholarship', which originally referred to a range of creative work, whose 'integrity was measured by the ability to think, communicate, and learn' (p. 15).

Scholarship, then, is certain habits of mind, and clinical scholarship modifies the noun only by focusing on observation in and of the work, including the perception of one's own participation in it (Diers 1995). To these observations are applied disciplined habits of analysis and analogy that are carefully styled and even more carefully modified so that, when written, the activity produces new understanding, new knowledge (Diers 1995). It would be demanding to advance on Nightingale's words about observation. "the trained power of attending to one's own impressions made by one's own sense, so that these should *tell* the nurse how a patient is, is the *sine quo non* of being a nurse at all" (Nightingale 1883, p. 1038). That said, nurses should revisit Nightingale's caution: "merely looking at the sick is not observing ... to look is not always to see" (p 1038). According to Diers (1995) to see is not always to notice, to recognise something observed (including felt by the emotional machinery) as different, a signal perhaps, and worth the process of reflection (Diers 1995).

Therefore, the term scholarship inhabits a broad place semantically, conceptually and in practice. 'Scholarship' signifies the principled space that connects integrity, research, teaching, learning, personal development and contribution to the world.

The term personifies the hermeneutic principle that the human mind must remain open, which is at the core of critical thinking and being. Scholarship is permeated by the principles of research: ethical, systematic enquiry that pushes the boundaries of what is possible to know. And scholarly enquiry, whatever its focus, needs to afford opportunities for critical engagement with the very structures within which these practices occur, and with the power relations that sustain them (Fung 2017, p. 105).

There are various terms in the literature interrelated with scholarship that warrant clarification. According to Boyer (1990) scholars are needed who not only skilfully explore the frontiers of knowledge, but also integrate ideas, connect thought to action, and inspire students. The very complexity of modern life requires more, not less, information; more, not less, participation (Boyer 1990). Further, Meleis (1992) describes a scholar as "a thinker, one who conceptualises the questions as well as pursues the answers" (p. 328), who sees the whole and how things fit within the larger view (Starck 1996). Besides, Diers (1995) cites Cardinal Newman (1852/1976), the hallmarks of the scholar are a scientific formation of mind, an acquired faculty of judgement, of clear sightedness, of sagacity, of wisdom, or philosophical reach of mind, and intellectual self-possession and repose acquired by discipline and habit. The enemies of scholarship would be fraud and deceit, superficiality and laziness, fuzziness of mind, lack of discipline, lack of respect for the observed world or the work of others (p. 25). According to Shulman (2000) a scholar is a consummate professional; an individual that continuously reflects on their practice while ensuring high standards, and who is open to advancing knowledge to others. For the advanced practice nursing practitioner to engage in the role of scholar using the dimensions of scholarship identified by Boyer would dictate they examine their own individual practice through reflection, investigation, expression and modify that practice and apply to that practice the same exacting standards of evaluation recommended by Glassick et al. (1997) (see Chaps. 3 and 6).

The "family of terms *scholarship-scholar-scholarly* point, on the one hand to the outcomes of research or intellectual work (she contributed greatly to *scholarship*; his *scholarly* output comprised hundreds). They also signify the qualities intrinsic in their way of working (his *scholarship* was evident from the start; she presented herself as suitably *scholarly* for the position). Finally, they identify intentions and goals (she devoted her life to *scholarship*), and they even manage to describe the person *as a person* (despite all it cost him, he was a true *scholar* to the end)" (Andresen 2000, p. 139). Scholarship is also a *knowledge* term. In each case of using the scholarship family, a statement is being made about *what* someone knows—knowing that or knowing how, it matters not—but is not merely limited to that. An extremely knowledgeable person is not necessarily a scholar (Andresen 2000). 'The scholarship family denotes to the quality of their knowledge. Thus, scholarship may not only concern their knowing itself (*what* they know) but also their approach to acquiring knowledge (their inquiry modes, or *ways* of knowing) and their means of advancing *or* disseminating knowledge (their mastery of teaching, writing, bibliography, taxonomy, rhetoric or public advocacy)' (Andresen 2000, p. 139).

1.2.2   Research and Scholarship Are Almost Synonymous

At scholarship's core lie the principles and practices of critical enquiry and dia-logue, directed simultaneously towards both the development of self *and* engage-ment with and impact on others. This engagement may range from 'service' to peers, the department or institution, to local/regional engagement with communi-ties, professions and organisations, to principled engagement at national, regional and international levels. Effective engagement is interactive: it is not just a unilateral dissemination of findings. It reflects that 'integrity' referred to by Boyer, 'measured by the ability to think, communicate, and learn' (Boyer 1990, p. 15). Boyer empha-sised that understanding scholarship exclusively as the scholarship of discovery or traditional research needed to be reconsidered. According to Boyer (1990) the time has come to move beyond the tired old "teaching versus research" debate and give the familiar and honourable term "scholarship" a broader, more capacious meaning, one that brings legitimacy to the full scope of academic work. Boyer went on to explain: surely, scholarship means engaging in original research. But the work of the scholar also means stepping back from one's investigation, looking for connec-tions, building bridges between theory and practice, and communicating one's knowledge effectively to students (Boyer 1990, p. 16). Within some disciplinary discourses, scholarship is tantamount to engaging competently in empirical research and then getting published in high-ranking journals. This makes a mockery of generic mission statements that promise to pursue "research, teaching and scholar-ship", as though scholarship were something distinct from research and teaching (Andresen 2000, p. 138). Scholarship is not simply a term of description. It is a term of recommendation, of challenge and it demands and expects something that can and should be accomplished in academic work, more than mere semantics (Boud 1990), as we engage in promoting a set of intellectual values contained within the meanings of the terms we articulate and use (Andresen 2000).

Specifically, Boyer concluded that the work of the professoriate might be thought of as having four separate, yet overlapping functions. These are: the scholarship of *discovery*; the scholarship of *integration*; the scholarship of *application*; and the scholarship of *teaching* (p. 16). The discovery of new knowledge through modes of inquiry associated with a given discipline with the goal of advancing the body of knowledge as it relates to the content of that discipline enables scholarship to be conceptualised more comprehensively, including next to the scholarship of discov-ery, the scholarship of teaching, application, and integration (Boyer 1990).

1.2.3   The Scholarship of Discovery

The scholarship of discovery is understood as original research that expands and or challenges current knowledge in a discipline. Boyer (1990) defined discovery as the creation of knowledge for knowledge sake; its purpose is to contribute not only to knowledge but also to the intellectual climate of academic institutions. Therefore, the scholarship of discovery is defined as the art of creating knowledge. According to Boyer, at its best it contributes not only to the stock of human knowledge but also to the intellectual climate of a college or university. Not just the outcomes, but the process, and especially the passion, give meaning to the effort (Boyer 1990, p. 17). Such scholarship also includes the creative work of scholars in the literary, visual and performing arts, hence the inclusion of all disciplines. Boyer's focus on the words 'process' and 'passion' identify the creative and absorbing nature of research. The question behind this kind of research is, 'What do I know and how do I know it?' This encompasses all aspects of research and investigation in all disciplines (McCarthy 2008, p. 10).

Thus, the probing mind of the researcher is a huge vital asset to the college/university and the world. Scholarly investigation, in all the disciplines, is at the very heart of academic life, and the pursuit of knowledge must be diligently cultivated and safeguarded. The intellectual excitement fuelled by this quest enlivens faculty and invigorates higher learning institutions, and in our complicated, vulnerable world, the discovery of new knowledge is absolutely crucial (Boyer 1990, p. 18).

The university as a social institution, however, is also more than the specific organisation where individual academic staff are employed and students earn their degrees. It is also a community of scholars each affiliated with certain disciplinary associations who play a major role in the extent to which the concept of a *scholarship of teaching* is valued within the discipline (Kreber 2003, p. 118).

1.2.4   The Scholarship of Teaching

Boyer's concept of a scholarship of teaching placed an important emphasis on extending the conception of teaching from transmission of knowledge to supporting transformative learning. In this sense, the scholarship of teaching involves stimulating active learning, critical thinking and commitment to life-long learning. Therefore, such a construction of knowledge transformation might then directly benefit society in an appropriate and opportune way, carefully captured by Boyer (1990) as "the work of the professor becomes consequential only as it is understood by others" (p. 30). This applies in the classroom but may also be understood as impacting on society as a whole (Peel 2009).

It is essential to distinguish between scholarly teaching and scholarship of teaching and learning, which can also be translated to all of the other dimensions of scholarship. Scholarship is about making scholarly processes transparent and publicly accessible for peer scrutiny. Trigwell and Shale (2004) use Andresen's (2000) ideas to describe a scholarly process as involving personal, but rigorous, intellectual development, inquiry and action built on values such as honesty, integrity, open-mindedness, scepticism and intellectual humility. Consequently, whilst teaching practice might be considered *scholarly* in that it is informed by personal research, and involves scientific inquiry and reflection into appropriate content, teaching methods and techniques, it can only, according to Shulman, then become *scholarship* once it is subject to peer review and publication:

We develop a scholarship of teaching when our work as teachers becomes public, peer-reviewed and critiqued, and exchanged with other members of our professional communities so they, in turn, can build on our work. These are the qualities of all scholarship (Shulman 2000, p. 50).

Making reference to the Scholarship of Teaching and Learning, Kanuka (2011) as a specialist in education questions whether Shulman's (2000) statement of the qualities of scholarship are, in fact, qualities of scholarship—or more precisely, enough to be considered as scholarly works in the educational research community. Is making our work 'public, peer-review and critiqued' sufficient to be considered as 'scholarship' in teaching and learning? Or is 'public, peer-review and critiqued' those characteristics that comprise a scholarly publication? (Kanuka 2011, p. 9). Since Boyer, a debate over the years has been the relation of scholarship of teaching and learning (SoTL) inquiry to theory and research on teaching and learning. SoTL brings together all the disciplines of higher education. That said, it is challenging to account for its epistemological stance, and to agree on the criteria that might bring consensus about the validity of any inquiry it generates (Fanghanel et al. 2015).

There is a need for *peer review* to cover all *aspects* of scholarly life—not only research but teaching and service as well. If teaching and service are aspects of scholarship, then surely the community of scholars have a stake in monitoring how well this scholarship is being performed. Or, to put the matter more bluntly according to Edgerton et al. (1991); when and if the scholarly communities apply peer review to teaching and service as they now do to research, then, and only then, will they have finally said, "We respect not only research but teaching and service as well" (p. 56). With this vision in mind, the advanced practice nursing practitioner should design their portfolio (see Chap. 6) in order to embrace the full range of their scholarly lifecycle. 'Whatever its size, or purpose, if you use the portfolio to build a *culture* of professionalism—professionalism in teaching, professionalism in research, and professionalism in service—you will be part of a noble understanding' (Edgerton et al. 1991, p. 56).

1.2.5 Scholarship of Integration

The scholarship of integration according to Boyer (1990) means making connections across disciplines, placing specialities in a larger context, in order to illuminate data in an enlightening way. Previously located on the margins of academic endeavour, the scholarship of integration is now central because it is definitely best equipped to respond to contemporary problems at both individual and societal level (Boyer 1990). Researchers are positioning their discovery work, or that of others, into broader intellectual patterns, thus moving beyond the disciplinary silos to build interdisciplinary partnerships with capacity to respond to complex human problems. This form of scholarship interprets and gives meaning to isolated facts and creates new perspectives that can answer questions not originally possible to answer (Pereyra-Rojas et al. 2017; Hofmeyer et al. 2007). The advanced practice nursing practitioner can engage in this intellectual activity with other disciplines as they ask the germane question; "what do the findings mean for nursing and is there a need to reconfigure the service and its impact on key stakeholders and in particular the recipients of the service?"

1.2.6   Scholarship of Application

Evaluating the scholarship of application is grounded on finding cases of applied scholarly activities and developing comprehensive reporting methods. According to Boyer (1990) there must be a direct correlation between the intellectual work of the scholar and the applied work, such as consultation analysis, and evaluation. Service is not a capture-all category, while social and civic projects are important, they should not be considered a part of the scholarship of application. What *should* be included are activities that relate directly to the intellectual work of the scholar and carried out through consultation, technical assistance, policy analysis, program evaluation, and the like (Boyer 1990, p. 37).

Consequently, reporting applied scholarship should contain the evaluation by the scholar, and by the recipients of the service, such as decision and policy makers and communities. Furthermore, the evaluation should include how the endeavour has not only benefited the community, but also added to the scholar's own understanding of their health sciences expertise (Hofmeyer et al. 2007). Boyer (1990) defines the scholarship of application as a dynamic process. In other words, this dimension of scholarship should not be interpreted as unidirectional in which discovered knowledge is merely applied. "New intellectual understandings can arise out of the very act of application" and this type of dynamic interaction revitalises theory and practice (Boyer 1990, p. 23),

According to Lyken-Segosebe (2017) within the disciplines of nursing and occupational therapy; the scholarship of practice is comparable to Boyer's (1990) scholarship of application, within the discipline of pharmacy; it occurs as Boyer's scholarship of application and Boyer's scholarship of engagement. The scholarship of practice is referred to by Burgener (2001) who argued that recognition and acceptance of the potential contributions of a broadened definition of scholarship, encompassing experiential ways of knowing, may assist in closing the existing gap between what is recognized and valued as scholarship in academic settings and the continuing unmet needs of the larger society (p. 48). Another option proposed by Diamond and Adam (2000) suggests that discipline specific scholarly work should be accepted as scholarship of practice if:

- The activity requires a high level of discipline-related expertise
- The activity breaks new ground, is innovative
- The activity can be replicated or elaborated
- The work and its results can be documented
- The work and its results can be peer reviewed
- The activity has significance or impact.

According to the AACN Position Statement on Defining Scholarship for the Discipline of Nursing: practice is conducted through the application of nursing and related knowledge to the assessment and validation of patient care outcomes, the measurement of quality life indicators, the development and refinement of practice protocols/strategies, the evaluation of systems of care, and the analysis of innovative health care delivery (AACN 1999).

Remaining active in nursing practice is also an essential part of nursing education by bringing state-of-the-art information to the lecture theatre and to the forefront of clinical practice and 'what matters most to the patient'. The nursing profession clearly engages in the scholarship of empirical research and publication, but there is a fundamental need for defining clinical practice with resultant applications and outcomes as nursing scholarship (Peterson and Stevens 2013). Therefore, the scholarship of practice seems to reside under the umbrella of the scholarship of application.

The literature infers that the scholarship of application and engagement are the same. Based on the definitions provided earlier, both scholarship of application and scholarship of engagement are relevant to the advanced practice nursing practitioner. Therefore, a cautionary note is emphasised that advanced practice nursing practitioners do not pay lip service to the scholarship of application/engagement dimension but strive to enact its ethos in its entirety as postulated by Boyer (1996). The enactment of the scholarship of application/engagement is through the design of and the commitment to 'communities of practice' that require buy-in, commitment and sustained resources from key stakeholders.

1.2.7   Scholarship of Engagement

Engaged scholarship refers to the relationship between the expertise and resources of the university and the systems of community to address social, ethical, and civic problems (Van De Ven and Johnson 2006). As Boyer puts it, universities and colleges remain the greatest sources of hope for intellectual and civic progress; therefore, the academy must become a more vigorous partner in the search for answers to our most pressing social, civic, moral, and economic problems (Pereyra-Rojas et al. 2017). According to Boyer (1996) the work of the academy ultimately must be directed toward larger, more humane ends and become more dynamically engaged in the issues of the day. Scholars uniquely gifted in research but also those who excel in the integration and application of knowledge, as well as those adept in the scholarship of teaching should be celebrated not restricted (Boyer 1990). Such a mosaic of talent, if acknowledged, would bring renewed vitality to higher learning and the nation (Boyer 1990, p. 27).

1.3   Framing the Scholarship of Engagement Within Communities of Practice

Studies of the practice of engaged scholarship in research intensive universities have found that community-engaged scholarship that is so needed in local and regional universities is "boundary-crossing"—it crosses disciplinary and functional boundaries (Cooper and Skipton 2013, p. 63). It therefore can manifest as engaged scholarship in research, engaged scholarship in teaching, and or engaged scholarship in professional service. It is scholarship guided by an engagement tenet that results in work connected in clear, thematic, and scholarly ways (Cooper and Skipton 2013). It offers a framework that has an explicit intention, the creation of connections between researchers/universities and practitioners/health care providers (McCormack 2011).

In a scholarship of engagement approach, the key is engaging *with* the community in outlining the purpose of the scholarship, in arriving at the questions driving the scholarship, and in the design, analysis, and dissemination of scholarship. In this cooperative creation of knowledge and problem-solving, community stakeholders (such as local businesses, provincial and municipal governments, non-governmental organisations and service users), faculty members, students, and staff are involved in framing the driving intellectual questions, in generating and interpreting the evidence, and in using the evidence for diverse purposes (Cooper and Skipton 2013). Moreover, engaged scholarship is not a one-time event. It is an ongoing process that requires institutional capacity, including individual leaders, leadership cadres, and an institutional unit that enables people to exchange information, learn from one another, and build mutual support (Checkoway 2013, p. 14). The distinctive and important contribution that faculty participants can make, i.e. scholarship then acts as the frame, it provides a stable architecture that enables faculty and students to collaborate with community stakeholders in ways that produce credible scholarship for enhanced public good and academic—research and student learning—outcomes (Cooper and Skipton 2013).

According to Sandman (2008), scholarship is *what* is being done, engaged scholarship is *how* it is done, and for the common or public good is *toward what end* it is done. Rather than simply responding to community or curricular needs, interests, problems, and requests in a just-in-time service-oriented mode, faculty become involved by framing their response as scholarship with the community constituents (Sandmann et al. 2000). This framing to simultaneously accomplish both school and community stakeholder objectives sets community-engaged research apart and promotes a practical and interdisciplinary approach most conducive to innovation (Cooper and Skipton 2013, p. 65).

Engaged scholarship implies a fundamental shift in how scholars define their relationships with the communities in which they are located, including other disciplines in the university and practitioners in relevant professional domains. Instead of viewing organisations as data collection sites and funding sources, an engaged scholar views them as a learning workplace where practitioners and scholars coproduce knowledge on important questions and issues by testing alternative ideas and different views of a common problem (Van De Ven and Johnson 2006, p. 809). According to Boyer (1990) academic researchers do not have the monopoly on knowledge creation. Abundant evidence shows that both the civic and academic health of any culture is vitally enriched as scholars and practitioners speak and listen carefully to each other (Boyer 1996, p. 15).

In particular, there remains a gap between what is known from research and the care that is provided in health systems. Reducing this know—do gap is one of the ethical imperatives of our time (Jull et al. 2017). One approach to bridging the know—do gap is to implement an interactive process of knowledge exchange between health researchers and knowledge users (Mitton et al. 2007). Knowledge exchange describes the interchange between research users and scientific producers (Mitton et al. 2007). The concept of knowledge exchange, therefore, encompasses all facets of knowledge production, sharing, storage, mobilisation, translation and use (Best and Holmes 2010). Moreover, Van De Ven and Johnson (2006) proposed a method of *engaged scholarship* in which researchers and practitioners coproduce knowledge that can advance the theory and practice in a given domain (p. 803).

The advanced practice nursing practitioner as an engaged scholar is ideally placed to undertake action research relevant to the policy context by giving due consideration to their legacy map and declared legacy/destination statement (see Chap. 6). This research methodology is referred to by Schon (1995, p. 27) as the new scholarship, new categories of scholarly activities. By exploiting differences in the kinds of knowledge that scholars and practitioners from diverse backgrounds bring to bear on a problem, engaged scholarship produces knowledge that is more penetrating and insightful than knowledge produced when scholars or practitioners work on a problem alone (Van De Ven and Johnson 2006, p. 802). Essentially engaged scholarship, irrespective of the particular methodology, can be considered to operate within a set of principles that utilises research processes that are negotiated and that are an integral component of the landscape of practice, whilst recognising that knowledge is contextually bound and therefore new knowledge is derived from an engagement with the context of practice (McCormack 2011, p. 117).

In a systematic review of the knowledge exchange literature relevant to the health sector Contandriopoulos et al. (2010) identified how knowledge exchange processes primarily occur at two complimentary levels. The first, termed autonomy makes reference to potential users of knowledge being typically sovereign in their capacity to mobilise knowledge and subsequently, modify their practices, so that knowledge producers and users of knowledge were considered as two independent groups. In contrast, Contandriopoulos et al. (2010) identified a second level at which knowledge exchange processes can occur, termed interdependency, with high levels of interconnectedness among all participants. The defining feature of this type of model is that participants do not have autonomy to translate scientific knowledge into practice independently (Cvitanovic et al. 2015).

The advanced practice nursing practitioner/aspirant needs to consider how to generate new understandings about practice utilising methodologies appropriate to foster critique of that practice. In other words, focus on an epistemology appropriate to scholarship that facilitates reflection in and on action (see Chap. 6). It must account for and legitimise not only the use of knowledge produced in the academy, but the practitioner's generation of actionable knowledge in the form of models or prototypes that can be carried over, by reflective transfer, to new practice situations, which includes what Kurt Lewin described as action research (Schon 1995, p. 34).

In order to legitimise the new scholarship, higher education institutions will have to learn organizationally to open up the prevailing epistemology so as to foster new forms of reflective action research that requires building up communities of inquiry capable of criticising such research and fostering its development (Schon 1995, p. 34). These learning communities are contexts within which knowledge production and professional practice and learning occur. The implication for advanced practice nursing doctoral and professional programs is that they should construct communities of practice within which those preparing for work as scholars or professionals can develop and experience opportunities to work with a variety of stakeholders and further develop their professional identities. That professional identity is a way of talking about how learning changes who the advanced practice nursing practitioner/aspirant is and creates personal histories of becoming in the context of their communities of practice. Generative and collaborative relationships between experienced scholars and those earlier in their career should characterise such learning communities (Austin and McDaniels 2016, p. 34). In order to sustain the vitality of higher education in our time, a new vision of scholarship is required, one dedicated not only to the renewal of the academy, but, ultimately, to the renewal of society itself (Boyer 1990 p. 81) and ultimately closer to the complicated and sometimes vulnerable world of clinical practice.

1.4   Conclusion

Scholarship is not simply a term of description. It is a term of recommendation, of challenge and it demands and expects something that can and should be accomplished in academic work, as practitioners engage in promoting a set of intellectual values contained within the meanings of the terms articulated and used on a daily basis. Five areas of scholarship; discovery, integration, application, teaching, and engagement were presented for consideration. The scholarship of discovery is defined as the art of creating knowledge. According to Boyer, at its best it contributes not only to the stock of human knowledge but also to the intellectual climate of a college or university. Not just the outcomes, but the process, and especially the passion, give meaning to the effort (Boyer 1990). Such scholarship also includes the creative work of scholars in the literary, visual and performing arts, hence the inclusion of all disciplines. Scholarly investigation, in all the disciplines, is at the very heart of academic life. The university as a social institution, however, is also more than the specific organisation where individual academic staff are employed and students earn their degrees. It is also a community of scholars. When and if the scholarly communities apply peer review to teaching and service as they now do to research, then, and only then, will they have finally said, "We respect not only research but teaching and service as well" (Edgerton et al. 1991, p. 56). With this vision in mind, the advanced practice nursing practitioner/aspirant should consider the landscape of their portfolio (see Chap. 6) in order to embrace the full range of their scholarly lifecycle.

The scholarship of integration interprets and gives meaning to isolated facts and creates new perspectives that can answer questions not originally possible to answer. The advanced practice nursing practitioner can engage in this intellectual activity with other disciplines as they ask the germane question; "what do the findings mean for nursing and is there a need to reconfigure the service and its impact on key stakeholders and in particular on those recipients of the service?"

Both scholarship of application and scholarship of engagement are relevant to the advanced practice nursing practitioner/aspirant. The literature infers that the scholarship of application and engagement are the same. That said, 'a community of practice' provides a platform for the enactment of the scholarship of engagement and setting up such a community requires not only committment but sustained resources from key stakeholders. Furthermore, it is through the process of individual pursuit of knowledge, sharing that knowledge and experiences with other groups that advanced practice nursing practitioners/aspirants learn from each other and have the opportunity to develop themselves personally and professionally (Wenger and Lave 1991). Engaged scholarship implies a fundamental shift in how scholars define their relationships with the communities in which they are located. Instead of seeing organisations as data collection sites and funding sources, an engaged scholar views them as a learning workplace where practitioners and scholars become co-producers of knowledge. According to Boyer (1990) academic researchers do not have the monopoly on knowledge creation. Abundant evidence shows that both the civic and academic health of any culture is vitally enriched as scholars and practitioners converse and listen carefully to each other (Boyer 1996).

Framing 'communities of practice' can become the operational lever for the enactment of the adapted dimensions of Boyer's scholarship, whereby advanced practice nursing practitioners co-produce knowledge with other disciplines on important questions by testing alternative views of a common problem using a methodology appropriate to that scholarship. The individual pursuit of knowledge is always situated in a social and cultural context in a community of practice that enables the advanced practice nursing practitioner/aspirant become part of a larger cohort of professionals, sharing a common pool of knowledge in clinical practice, while advancing nursing's own body of knowledge encapsulated within that inter-professional scholarly experience.

References

American Association of Colleges of Nursing. Position statement on defining scholarship for the discipline of nursing. 1999. Accessed from http://www.aacn.nche.edu/publications/position/defining-scholarship.

Andresen L. A useable, trans-disciplinary conception of scholarship. High Educ Res Dev. 2000;19:137–53.

Austin A, McDaniels M. Impact on doctoral and professional education. In: Moser D, Todd R, Braxton J, Associates, editors. Scholarship reconsidered. San Francisco, CA: Jossey Bass; 2016. p. 31–9.

Best A, Holmes B. Systems thinking, knowledge and action: towards better models and methods. Evid Pol. 2010;6:145–59.

Boud D. Assessment and the promotion of academic values. Stud High Educ. 1990;15:101–11.

Boyer E. Scholarship reconsidered: priorities of the professoriate. Carnegie Foundation for the Advancement of Teaching. Princeton, NJ: Princeton University Press; 1990.

Boyer E. The scholarship of engagement. J Pub Serv Outreach. 1996;1:11–20.

Burgener S. Scholarship of practice for a practice profession. J Prof Nurs. 2001;17:46–54.

Canadian Association of Schools of Nursing. Scholarship among nursing faculty: position statement, Ottawa. 2013. Accessed from http://www.casn.ca/wp-content/uploads/2014/10/ScholarshipinNursingNov2013ENFINALmm.pdf.

Checkoway B. Strengthening the scholarship of engagement in higher education. J High Educ Outreach Engag. 2013;17:7–21.

Cooper T, Skipton M. Revisiting the mission of the business school through scholarship of engagement. J High Educ Theor Pract. 2013;13:57–71.

Contandriopoulos D, Lemire M, Denis L, Tremblay E. Knowledge exchange process in organisations and policy arenas: a narrative systematic review of the literature. MillBank Quart. 2010;88:444–83.

Cvitanovic C, Hobday A, van Kerhoff L, Wilson S, Dobbs K. Improving knowledge exchange among scientists and decision-makers to facilitate the adaptive governance of marine resources: a review of knowledge and research needs. Ocean Coast Manag. 2015;112:25–35.

Diamond R, Adam B. The disciplines speak: rewarding the scholarly professional, and creative work of faculty. Washington DC: American Association for Higher Education; 2000.

Diers D. Clinical scholarship. J Prof Nurs. 1995;11:24–30.

Ding A. Challenging scholarship: a thought piece. Language Scholar. 2016. Accessed from http://languagescholar.leeds.ac.uk/. ISSN:2398-8509.

Edgerton R. Foreword. In: Meara K, Rice R, editors. Faculty priorities reconsidered: rewarding multiple forms of scholarship. San Francisco, CA: Jossey Bass; 2005.

Edgerton R, Hutchings P, Quinlan K. The teaching portfolio: capturing the scholarship of teaching. Washington, DC: American Association for Higher Education; 1991.

Fanghanel J, McGowen S, Parker P, McConnel LC, Potter J, Locke W, Healey M. Literature review. Defining and supporting the scholarship of teaching and learning (SoTL): a sector-wide study. York: Higher Education Academy; 2015.

Fung D. Strength-based scholarship and good education: the scholarship circle. Innov Educ Teach Int. 2017;54:101–10.

Glassick C, Huber M, Maeroff G. Scholarship assessed-evaluation of the professoriate. San Francisco, CA: Jossey-Bass; 1997.

Hofmeyer A, Newton M, Scott C. Valuing the scholarship of integration and the scholarship of application in the academy for health science scholars: recommended methods. BioMed Central. 2007;5:5. https://doi.org/10.1186/1478-4505-5.5.

Jull J, Giles A, Graham I. Community-based participatory research and integrated knowledge translation: advancing the co-creation of knowledge. Implement Sci. 2017;12:150. https://doi.org/10.1186/s.13012-017-0696-3.

Kanuka H. Keeping the scholarship in the scholarship of teaching and learning. Int J Scholar Teach Learn. 2011;5:3. https://doi.org/10.20429/ijsotl.2011.050103.

Kielhofner G. A scholarship of practice: creating discourse between theory, research and practice. In: Crist P, Kielhofner G, editors. The scholarship of practice: academic practice collaborations for promoting occupational therapy. New York, NY: Haworth Press; 2005a. p. 7–16.

Kielhofner G. Research concepts in clinical scholarship---scholarship and practice: bridging the divide. Am J Occup Ther. 2005b;59:231–9.

Kreber C. The scholarship of teaching: a comparison of conceptions held by experts and regular academic staff. High Educ. 2003;46:93–121.

Lyken-Segosebe D. The scholarship of practice. Appl Discip. 2017;178:21–33.

Meleis A. On the way to scholarship: from master's doctorate. J Prof Nurs. 1992;8:328–34.

Mitton C, Adair C, McKenzie E, Patten S, Perry B. Knowledge transfer and exchange: review and synthesis of the literature. MilBank Quart. 2007;85:729–68.

McCarthy M. The scholarship of teaching and learning in higher education: an overview. In: Murray R, editor. The scholarship of teaching and learning in higher education. Maidenhead: Open University Press; 2008. p. 6–15.

McCormack B. Engaged scholarship and research impact: integrating the doing and using of research in practice. J Res Nurs. 2011;16:111–27.

Newland J, Truglio-Londrigan M. Faculty practice: facilitation of clinical integrations into the academic triad model. J Prof Nurs. 2003;19:269–78.

Newman CJH. In: Ker IT, editor. The idea of a university. Oxford: Clarendon Press; 1852/1976.

Nightingale F. Nurses: thinking of. In: Quain R, editor. Quain's dictionary of medicine. 5th ed. New York, NY: Appleton; 1883. p. 1038–41.

Peel D. Embracing scholarship in the built environment. J Educ Built Environ. 2009;4:1–8.

Pereyra-Rojas M, Mu E, Gaskin J, Lingham T. The higher organisational-scholar tension: how scholarship compatibility and the alignment of organisational and faculty skills, values and support affects scholar's performance and well-being. Front Psych. 2017;8:450. https://doi.org/10.3389/psyg.2017.00450.

Peterson K, Stevens J. Integrating the scholarship of practice into the nurse academician portfolio. Nurs Fac Publ Pap. 2013;1. Accessed from http://digitalcommons.brockport.edu/nursing_facpub/1.

Sandmann L, Foster-Fishman P, Lloyd J, Rosaen C. Managing critical tensions how to strengthen the scholarship component of outreach. Change. 2000;32:44–52.

Sandman L. Conceptualisation of the scholarship of engagement in higher education: a strategic review, 1996-2006. J High Educ Outreach Engag. 2008;12:91–104.

Schon D. Knowing-in-action: the new scholarship requires a new epistemology. Change. 1995;27:27–34.

Shulman L. Teacher development: roles of domain expertise and pedagogical knowledge. J Appl Dev Psychol. 2000;21:129–35.

Starck P. Boyer's multidimensional nature of scholarship: a new framework for schools of nursing. J Prof Nurs. 1996;12:268–76.

Trigwell K, Shale S. Student learning and the scholarship of university teaching. Stud High Educ. 2004;29:523–36.

Van De Ven A, Johnson P. Knowledge for theory and practice. Acad Manage Rev. 2006;31:802–21.

Wenger E, Lave J. Situated learning: legitimate peripheral participation. Cambridge: Cambridge University Press; 1991.

Boyer's Pillars of Scholarship

2

2.1 Introduction

The pillars of scholarship are addressed in-depth: Scholarship of Discovery, Engagement, Teaching, Integration, and Application. The pillars of Boyer's scholarship are viewed as dynamic and interact forming an interdependent mosaic that can ground the scholarly activity of the advanced practice nursing practitioner/aspirant. Five principles related to the domains of scholarship are examined that foster strategies to connect a spirit of inquiry with the wider community. The Scholarship of Practice is placed in context. Clinical Scholarship is explored in the context of various definitions and its embeddedness within advanced practice nursing.

2.2 Context of Boyer's Pillars of Scholarship

Boyer (1990) defined scholarship as having at least four domains: discovery, engagement, teaching, integration, and application. The scholarship of discovery reflects the excitement of a new idea, the exhilaration of a new insight, and the search for knowledge for the joy of knowing. Outcomes of such research abound in refereed journals. However, the scholarship of discovery is not the mere accumulation of publications to satisfy the "counters" of vita lines at tenure and promotion time (Atkinson 2001, p. 1220). That said, the challenge for the scholar with respect to the scholarship of discovery is to develop a coherent program of research while meeting the needs of the agency (Jacelon et al. 2010). The advanced practice nursing practitioner/aspirant can commence engagement with the process of developing a career legacy map portfolio (see Chap. 6), which can be a starting point that inter sects across all of the dimensions of Boyer's scholarship, paving the way for grounding their practice in nursing theoretical perspectives (Chinn and Falk-Rafael 2018).

© Springer Nature Switzerland AG 2019   17
L. O'Connor, *The Nature of Scholarship, a Career Legacy Map and Advanced Practice*, Advanced Practice in Nursing, https://doi.org/10.1007/978-3-319-91695-8_2

2.2.1   The Scholarship of Discovery

The first and most familiar element in our model, the *scholarship of discovery*, comes closest to what is meant when academics speak of "research" (Boyer 1990, p. 17). The academy holds no tenet in higher regard than the pursuit of knowledge for its own sake, a fierce determination to give free rein to fair and honest inquiry, wherever it may lead (Boyer 1990). At its best, the scholarship of discovery contributes not only to the stock of human knowledge but also to the intellectual climate of a college or university; the process, the outcomes, and especially the passion of discovery enhance the meaning of the effort and of the institution itself (Glassick et al. 1997, p. 9). Through research, universities simply must continue to push back the frontiers of human knowledge (Boyer 1996, p. 16).

Fung (2017) positions the question; if good education is categorised by inquiry and critique directed at both the development of individuals and the public good, how might research, 'the scholarship of discovery', be characterised? Research has been defined as 'advancing the frontiers of knowledge' (Nurse 2015, p. 11): so how does it relate then to education and to scholarship more broadly? (Fung 2017, p. 105). Research is a valuable and prestigious commodity. But a value-based conception of research connects health care professionals to the roots of scholarship in the round: ethical inquiry, application, communication and engagement, for the good of society. This translates to revisiting the purpose and values underpinning research, construed as a public good and not primarily a marker of esteem in the 'prestige economy' (Blackmore 2016), and may help both individuals and institutions reconsider the balance of their activities and goals (Fung 2017, p. 105).

Over the past two decades nurses have put intensive efforts into the scholarship of discovery. Every nursing student at the baccalaureate, master's, and doctoral level is well versed in the importance of research-based practice, the structure and process of continuing to discover new knowledge for the discipline (Starck 1996, p. 269). According to the AACN position statement, "the scholarship of discovery is the inquiry that produces the disciplinary and professional knowledge that is at the very heart of academic pursuits" (American Association of Colleges of Nursing 1999). It entails how the practitioner uses client and family as participants in exploring clinical questions (Peterson and Stevens 2013). Furthermore, advanced practice nursing practitioners/aspirants learn every day, what works and what does not in each individual nurse-patient encounter. In that encounter, nursing theoretical viewpoints supported and enriched by research guide them to be attentive, forensic, and responsive to the uniqueness of the situation and to the human person in that care context.

2.2.2   Scholarship of Engagement

Boyer suggested that the work of individual scholars, as researchers, has continued to be highly prized, and that also, in recent years, teaching has increasingly become more highly regarded, a cause for celebration. But he also believed that in many institutions of higher learning, the historic commitment to the "scholarship of engagement" dramatically declined (Boyer 1996, p. 13). Hence, the academy must become a more vigorous partner in the search for answers to our most pressing social, civic, economic, and moral problems, and must affirm its historic commitment to what he called the scholarship of engagement rather than "being viewed as a place where students get credentialed and faculty get tenured" (Boyer 1996, p. 14).

In *Scholarship Reconsidered*, Boyer called not only for the scholarship of discovering knowledge, the scholarship of integrating knowledge to avoid pedantry, and the sharing of knowledge to avoid discontinuity, but also for the application of knowledge, to avoid irrelevance (Boyer 1990). In addition, when applying knowledge, this does not mean "doing good", although that's important, but by scholarship of application we mean having professors become what Donald Schon (1995) called "reflective practitioners", moving from theory to practice, and from practice back to theory, which in fact makes theory, then, more authentic—something we're learning in education and medicine, in law and architecture, and all the rest (Boyer 1996, p. 17). In addition, and incidentally, by making knowledge useful, we mean everything from building better bridges to building better lives, which involves not only the professional schools but the arts and sciences as well (Boyer 1996).

The term civic engagement refers to collective actions that people take to create changes in a community or society (Checkoway 2013). Then, campuses would be viewed by both students and professors not as isolated islands, but as staging grounds for action. But at a deeper level, ultimately, the scholarship of engagement also means creating a special climate in which the academic and civic cultures communicate continuously and creatively with each other, helping to enlarge what anthropologist Clifford Geertz described as the universe of human discourse and enriching the quality of life for all of us (Boyer 1996, p. 20). Moreover, Burrage et al. (2005) assert that embracing the scholarship of engagement will aid in the attainment of scholarly and professional goals of nurse faculty and non-academic partners such as groups of patients and practice-focussed nurses. Thus, nurses' contribution as scholars will be more substantial and meaningful to communities and nursing practice, and the utilisation of knowledge will result in more timely and useful interventions (p. 223).

A scoping review undertaken by Beaulieu et al. (2018) reported that faculty are uniquely positioned at the heart of the engagement process, at the interface between both society and academia, with three main functions: teaching, research, and service. Furthermore, to foster connections with society, faculty must adhere to five principles: (1) high-quality scholarship; (2) reciprocity; (3) identified community needs; (4) boundary-crossing; and (5) democratization of knowledge (Beaulieu et al. 2018, p. 13). The five aforementioned principles can be applied in faculty's ways of doing research, engaging in community service, and teaching by building links between the university and society, science and practice, and research and action. The university as an institution plays a major role in implementing engaged scholarship, in particular by providing a clear mission, a structure that recognises and rewards engagement activities, logistical support for engagement projects, and support for students who wish to become engaged (Beaulieu et al. 2018).

Furthermore, Boyer described the emergence of a "new" stream in the academic world, engaged scholarship (e.g., engaged teaching, engaged research, engaged service), still perceived today as a promising avenue both for increasing the university's legitimacy and for addressing the knowledge-to-action gap.

2.2.3 Scholarship of Teaching

Teaching is also a dynamic endeavour involving all the analogies, metaphors, and images that build bridges between the teacher's understanding and the student's learning (Boyer 1990, p. 23). Good teaching means that faculty, as scholars, are also learners, teaching, at its best, means not only transmitting knowledge, but *transforming* and *extending* it as well (Boyer 1990, p. 24).

Trigwell et al. (2000) postulate that university teachers must be informed of the theoretical perspectives and literature of teaching and learning in their discipline, and be able to collect and present rigorous evidence of their effectiveness, from these perspectives, as teachers, which in turn, involves reflection, inquiry, evaluation, documentation and communication (p. 156). Therefore, according to Trigwell et al. (2000) the aim of scholarly teaching is simple: it is to make transparent how we have made learning possible.

One of the ideas embedded in the scholarship of teaching and learning is for teachers in higher education to go public with lessons from their pedagogical work. In a brief but powerful article in *Change* magazine, Shulman (1993) suggested that teaching has low status in the academy because it is typically treated in a way that "removes it from the community of scholars" (p. 6). He offered a threefold prescription (Huber 2009, p. 2). First, teaching in higher education needs to be (re)connected to communities that matter, especially the disciplines. Second, in order to become community property, teaching would have "to be made visible through artefacts that capture its richness and complexity" (pp. 6–7). Finally, instead of relying solely on student evaluations, teaching should be reviewed-and judged-by "communities of peers beyond the office next door" (Huber 2009, p. 2). Some of the aforementioned prescriptions identified by Shulman have resonance for all the dimensions of Boyer's scholarship and advanced practice nursing practitioners/aspirants should give due consideration to each of them and their translation within and across their scholarly activities.

The AACN position statement clearly outlines and describes ways in which the scholarship of teaching can be conducted by nurses by focusing on the teaching-learning process, the development of innovative teaching and evaluation methods, program development, learning outcome evaluation, and professional role modelling (AACN 1999). Reflection is considered an important part of the process. Kreber and Cranton (2000) proposed that individuals who practice the scholarship of teaching engage in reflection on existing knowledge about teaching and learning generated through research as well as in reflection on their personal or experience-based knowledge teaching. Andresen (2000) argued that scholarship, including the scholarship of teaching, should be inquiry-driven, involve critical reflectivity, and scrutiny by peers. This way of conceptualising the notion of a scholarship of teaching, therefore, is activity oriented.

According to Trigwell and Shale (2004) without a *discourse* of teaching it would be almost impossible to enhance teaching expertise; excellence in teaching discourse, and excellence in the teaching that enables students to learn, are two different things (p. 527). Excellence in teaching is usually identified on the basis of a judgement made about *performance* (Kreber 2002, p. 9). Faculty, according to Bereiter and Scardamalia (1993) who continuously engage in self-regulating their learning about teaching develop expertise in teaching. In contrast, teachers who at one point engaged in reflection and as a consequence developed a repertoire of effective algorithms, strategies, or routines they rely on exclusively, would, according to the literature on expertise, most likely not be considered experts though some may indeed be "effective teachers" or "excellent teachers" (Kreber 2002, p. 13). Experts are excellent teachers, but excellent teachers are *not necessarily* experts (Kreber 2002, p. 13). Of note, a scholarship of teaching is *not* synonymous with excellent teaching, it requires a kind of "going meta," in which faculty frame and systematically investigate questions related to student learning—the conditions under which it occurs, what it looks like, how to deepen it, and do so with an eye not only to improving their own classroom but to advancing practice beyond it (Hutchings and Shulman 1999). This conception of the scholarship of teaching is not something we presume all faculty (even the most excellent and scholarly teachers among them) will or should do, though it would be good to see that more of them have the opportunity to do so if they wish (Hutchings and Shulman 1999, pp. 13–14). For Pinar, taking a value-based, critical stance in his work on curriculum stated that teachers are 'communicants in a complicated conversation' (Pinar 2012, p. 25). Pinar argues that good education is not about teachers' facilitating learning but about giving both teachers and students a voice:

> Expressing one's subjectivity through academic knowledge is how … one demonstrates to students that scholarship can speak to them, how in fact scholarship can enable them to speak (Pinar 2012, p. 22).

Consequently, Fung questions how 'good' education might be defined? Through one lens, it is the efficient meeting of one's own 'measurable objectives' in such a way that comparable standards of 'quality', 'achievement' and 'accountability' can be recognised. Through another lens, it is the 'becoming' of individuals and communities through dialogue and engagement, leading to the advancement of shared human principles. Therefore, lens one may be operationally useful, but the second lens exemplifies more fully the integrity and purposes of that scholarship (Fung 2017, p. 104).

Trigwell et al. (2000) offer a model for making transparent the process of making learning possible. The model has four dimensions relating to the areas (a) being informed about teaching and learning generally and in the teachers' own discipline; (b) reflection on that information, the teachers' particular context and the relations between the two; (c) the focus of the teaching approach adopted; and (d) communication of the relevant aspects of the other three dimensions to members of the community of scholars (p. 167). All four dimensions are considered to be a necessary part of the scholarship of teaching, the model makes use of the inclusive hierarchy of categories from results of an empirical study to illustrate qualitatively different approaches to the scholarship of teaching. Teachers can be engaged in scholarly teaching practices in the sense that they include aspects of all four dimensions described in the model, other teachers, who engage in these same practices but qualitatively go beyond them in one or more dimensions, would be considered to be adopting a more inclusive approach to the scholarship of teaching (Trigwell et al. 2000, p. 167).

Boyer made a case that the scholarship of teaching be aligned with the scholarships of integration and application and equal in importance to the scholarship of discovery. He focused primarily on scholarly teaching and argued that engaged teaching is an enticement to scholarship and a link between other scholarships and student learning (Beach 2016).

2.2.4   Scholarship of Integration

This dimension of scholarship involves stepping back from a narrow area of research to search for connections between discoveries obtained by different approaches or even from varied disciplines. It involves faculty members in overcoming the isolation and fragmentation of discipline specific silos. The scholarship of integration makes connections within and between disciplines, altering the contexts in which people view knowledge and balancing the inclination to split knowledge into ever more obscure fragments. Often, the scholarship of integration educates non-specialists by giving meaning to isolated facts and putting them in perspective. Moreover, the scholarship of integration is serious, disciplined work that seeks to interpret, draw together, and bring new insight to bear on original research (Glassick et al. 1997, p. 9). Further Boyer (1990) defined the scholarship of integration as "giving meaning to isolated facts, putting them in perspective…making connections across the disciplines, placing specialities in larger contexts, illuminating data in a revealing way, and educating non-specialists" (p. 18). The scholarship of integration is work that compiles, interprets, and generates new insights from original research (Boyer 1990; Beattie 2000). An example of integrative scholarship could be writing textbooks, especially if their point is to synthesise, provide conceptual frameworks and elaborate a sociological understanding of the world (Atkinson 2001, p. 1220).

The scholarship of integration occurs when nursing interacts with other disciplines to complete analysis of health policy, development of interdisciplinary educational programs and service projects, integrative reviews of the literature, and models or paradigms across disciplines (AACN 1999). This scholarship suggests that the researcher as teacher needs to ask the question, 'How can the findings be interpreted in ways that provide a larger, more comprehensive understanding?' as Boyer pointed out that the scholarship of integration is closely related to that of discovery. It involves, first, 'doing research at the boundaries where fields converge' (1990, p. 19). Such work is according to Boyer (1990) increasingly important as traditional disciplinary categories prove confining, forcing new typologies of knowledge (Boyer 1990).

Advanced practice nursing practitioners are in a primary locus to communicate with colleagues in other fields, and discover patterns that connect their own research or the research of other disciplines into larger intellectual patterns. Such efforts are increasingly essential since specialisation, without broader perspective, risks pedantry, the distinction we are drawing here between "discovery" and "integration" can be best understood, perhaps, by the questions posed (Boyer 1990, p. 19). Those engaged in discovery ask, "What is to be known, what is yet to be found?" Those engaged in integration ask, "What do the findings mean? Is it possible to interpret what's been discovered in ways that provide a larger, more comprehensive understanding?" Questions such as these call for the power of critical analysis and interpretation (Boyer 1990, p. 19). They have a legitimacy of their own and if carefully pursued can lead the scholar from information to knowledge and even, to wisdom (Boyer 1990, p. 20).

2.2.5   Scholarship of Application

The next element, the scholarship of application, moves toward engagement as the scholar asks, "How can knowledge be responsibly applied to consequential problems?" (Glassick et al. 1997, p. 9). Lessons learned in the application of knowledge can enrich teaching, and new intellectual understandings can arise from the very act of application, such as in medical diagnosis, or study of a design defect in architecture and theory and practice interact in such ventures and improve each other (Glassick et al. 1997, p. 9).

In application scholarship, health science scholars build bridges and collaborative relationships with other disciplines, decision and policy makers and communities in order to apply theory to solve every-day problems (Hall 2001). The scholarship of application is applied research that is also engaged and is a dynamic process through which theory and practice interact. In the process of applying what we know, we also discover new knowledge and thereby contribute to our knowledge base. Of note, doing the "housework" of the academy (committee work and other service) and "good citizenship" are not applied scholarship (Atkinson 2001, p. 1220).

The scholar uses his/her knowledge as a researcher and expertise as an advanced practice nursing practitioner to engage in organisation activity, as application is clearly germane to the landscape of practice. According to Peterson and Stevens (2013) nursing faculty engage in the scholarship of application in a variety of ways including advanced clinical practice, staff development, clinical problem solving, and consultation work. The scholarship of application is discipline specific and may not result in a product in the traditional sense of the word, but may result in products that allow for practice application such as policy development, practice protocols, care pathways or manuals (Peterson and Stevens 2013). This aspect of scholarship basically asks how knowledge can be used in a practical situation. The *application* of knowledge moves towards engagement as the scholar asks. "How can knowledge be responsibly applied to individuals as well as institutions?" And further, "Can social problems *themselves* define an agenda for scholarly investigation?" (Boyer 1990, p. 21).

The scholarship of *application*, is not a one-way street, the term itself may be misleading if it suggests that knowledge is first "discovered" and then "applied", the process is far more dynamic (Boyer 1990, p. 23). New intellectual understandings can arise out of the very act of application-whether in medical/nursing diagnosis, serving clients in psychotherapy, shaping public policy, creating architectural design, or working with the public schools. In activities such as these, theory and practice vitally interact, and one renews the other (Boyer 1990, p. 23). Clearly, the processes involved in application and engagement bring a more concrete and fluid aspect to the broad understanding of scholarship by demonstrating the dynamic interplay among all its components (Simpson 2000).

2.2.6   Scholarship of Practice

Boyer's ideas have made important contributions to discussions of how to prepare doctoral and professional students for careers in discovering new knowledge, engaging with an array of learners, improving teaching and learning experiences in their fields, connecting knowledge from within and across different disciplines, and addressing the challenging problems confronting humankind at this time in our history (Austin and McDaniels 2016). Furthermore, the dynamism of the contexts within which doctoral students work requires a different type of scholar than was previously produced by doctoral programs: one strongly anchored in the scholarship of practice across disciplines (McDaniels and Skogsberg 2017, p. 73). The scholarship of practice is a type of research that aims to improve professional performance of individuals who implement that scholarship and build a knowledge base on efficacious professional practices to help institutional and societal leaders in the academy, industry, and the public sectors (Braxton 2005). Therefore, preparing graduate students with the foundational competences to engage in a variety of professional practices is not enough; McDaniels and Skogsberg (2017) also recommend introducing doctoral students to, and having them engage in, a type of reflection known as the *scholarship of practice* (p. 73). This approach to scholarship requires an adjustment of the traditional view of researcher driven science to a view of collaboration between the scholar and the community (Burrage et al. 2005). In this view, the university and the faculty member benefit by gaining access to research populations and clinical problems, whereas the community benefits by the opportunity to work closely with faculty to address community issues and learn how to enhance practice (Jacelon et al. 2010).

Society needs transdisciplinary professionals ready to collaborate with individuals in other fields to conceptualise across theoretical perspectives and multiple levels at the outset of their scientific experience (Nash 2008). The term *transdisciplinary* is used to refer to contexts both inside and outside the academy within which today's doctoral students will work—settings that reveal some of the very real and seemingly intractable challenges (McDaniels and Skogsberg 2017). According to Thompson (2009) creating cross-disciplinary research alliances is important as it is likely that this sort of research perspective is better suited to addressing the complex health issues encountered by patients, families and communities, but it is important that the nursing contribution is clear, valued and visible (p. 696). Scholarly collaboration between advanced practice nursing practitioners/aspirants, the academy and the community while unlocking discipline specific silos and keeping the nursing contribution on the agenda could note Kreindler et al. (2012) guiding questions. Kreindler et al. (2012) conducted a review of 300 research reports pertinent to professional socialisation and how educational and practice environments encourage or suppress the enactment of a patient-centered identity and offered the following guiding questions for health care leaders confronting the problem of silos:

1. Who are the relevant groups, and what are their relationships? How social identity might be playing a role in current organisational problems or conflicts?
2. Which groups need to be around the table to develop new ways of working? Can they come together immediately, or does intergroup tension necessitate that they first work separately?
3. Which identities matter most to participants, and how can these be mobilised? What change messages (and messengers) will fit the values and attributes cherished by each group?
4. What is the potential for context change? How might day-to-day factors that reinforce silos and conflict be replaced by others that promote more cooperative and equal interactions?
5. As change proceeds, how can identity threat (to valued groups' existence, status, distinctiveness, values,) be minimised? (p. 366).

These guiding questions are points for reflection prior to engaging with key stakeholders (see Chap. 6) and are pertinent to a scholarship of practice that could be partici patory and also transdisciplinary, led by advanced practice nursing practitioners/aspirants. Then the intellectual activity of thinking, analysis and synthesis becomes part of the medley of talent an advanced practice nursing practitioner/aspirant draws on in their scholarly accomplishments in the context of clinical practice. Actually, McDaniels and Skogsberg (2017) postulate that doctoral students must see their own disciplinary epistemologies objectively as only one of many legitimate knowledge sources and even as knowledge sources with limitations. This will enable doctoral students to be more open to the existence of legitimate professional practices and scholarship on topics they might have intuitively felt were important but perhaps viewed as "soft" or not as rigorous as ideas in their own fields (McDaniels and Skogsberg 2017, pp. 74–75).

2.3   Clinical Scholarship

It is easier to discuss what clinical scholarship is not than what it is. It is not mere journalistic reporting nor even the traditional case study, although clinical scholarship begins, as does clinical research, with observation, it builds differently (Diers

1995, p. 28). Clinical research begins with a curiosity; clinical scholarship with the sense of wonder that we call "marvel" (Diers 1995, p. 28). Simply feeling, intuiting, is not scholarship without informed, intelligent, and clinically grounded analysis. In research, attention is paid to the numbers or concepts; in scholarship, care with the language is critical. In both cases, the activity is not complete until it is written down (Diers 1995, p. 28). Excellent clinical research and scholarship share another potential similarity: 'they turn conventional ways of thinking upside down' (Diers 1995, p. 28).

An important contribution by Andresen (2000) is pertinent to the advanced practice nursing practitioner/aspirant and clinical scholarship and scholarly work. Three characteristics have now been identified as a starting point that could be useful tests by which scholarship and scholarly activities may be distinguishable from non-scholarly or less-than-scholarly. Whether they turn out to be sufficient and/or necessary will be something for ongoing argument to establish

1. Critical reflectivity as a sensibility, *a habit of mind*;
2. Scrutiny by peers, which is what publication permits as a *modus operandi*; and
3. Inquiry, as a *motivation* or *drive* (Andresen 2000, p. 141).

First, the quality of mind present in the person or represented by a scholar's work is one of critical reflectivity (Andresen 2000). Critical reflectivity captures a complex set of values such as integrity, open-mindedness, breadth combined with depth, scepticism, fairness, generosity, and intellectual humility and operate at two levels; commitment to effectively guide day-to-day matters in academic work and are open to public scrutiny and challenge (Andresen 2000, p. 140). Furthermore, Andresen (2000) postulates that scholarship invokes the notion of a "college of scholarly practitioners" and scholarly knowing, about anything whatsoever, is never final, but always subject to public scrutiny, discussion, reconsideration, and response to the challenge presented by the values already mentioned; an ethic of inquiry (p. 141).

2.4   Conclusion

Boyer's seminal work, "*Scholarship Reconsidered*" (1990) suggested that faculty should let go of the tired old research vs. teaching argument and focus on the idea that scholarship exists in all aspects of academic work and suggested there are at least four separate, but interdependent areas of scholarship. The scholarship of discovery reflects the excitement of a new idea, the exhilaration of a new insight, and the search for knowledge for the joy of knowing. Ultimately, the scholarship of engagement means creating a special climate in which the academic and civic cultures communicate continuously and creatively with each other. Reflection is considered an important part of the process of scholarly activity. Kreber and Cranton (2000) proposed that individuals who practice the scholarship of teaching engage in reflection on existing knowledge about teaching and learning generated through research as well as in reflection on their personal or experience-based knowledge teaching. Of note, experts are excellent teachers, but excellent teachers are *not necessarily* experts (Kreber 2002). A scholarship of teaching is *not* synonymous with excellent teaching, it requires a kind of "going meta," (Hutchings and Shulman 1999).

The scholarship of integration involves faculty members overcoming the isolation and fragmentation of the discipline specific silos. The scholarship of integration occurs when nursing interacts with other disciplines. Advanced practice nursing practitioners are in a primary locus to communicate with colleagues in other fields, and discover patterns that connect their own research or the research of other disciplines into larger intellectual patterns. Moreover, the processes involved in application and engagement bring a more concrete and fluid aspect to the broad understanding of scholarship by demonstrating the dynamic interplay among all its components. That said, society needs transdisciplinary professionals ready to collaborate with individuals in other fields to conceptualise across theoretical perspectives across multiple levels at the outset of their scientific experience. However, preparing graduate students with the foundational competences to engage in a variety of professional practices is not enough; it is also recommended introducing doctoral students to, and having them engage in, a type of reflection known as the scholarship of practice (McDaniels and Skogsberg 2017). The scholarship of practice is a type of research that aims to improve professional performance of individuals who implement that scholarship and build a knowledge base on efficacious professional practices to help institutional and societal leaders in the academy, industry, and the public sectors (Braxton 2005).

An important contribution by Andresen (2000) is pertinent to the advanced practice nursing practitioner/aspirant framing their clinical scholarship and scholarly work and are presented as a starting point; critical reflectivity as a sensibility, scrutiny by peers, and an ethic of inquiry, that will act as a powerful generator for enacting Boyer's scholarship domains (see Fig. 4.1) in the milieu of a comunity of inquiry.

References

American Association of Colleges of Nursing. Position statement on defining scholarship for the discipline of nursing. 1999. Accessed from http://www.aacn.nche.edu/publications/position/defining-scholarship.

Andresen L. A useable, transdisciplinary conception of scholarship. High Educ Res Dev. 2000;19:137–53.

Atkinson M. The scholarship of teaching and learning: reconceptualising scholarship and transforming the academy. Soc Forces. 2001;79:1217–29.

Austin A, McDaniels M. Impact on doctoral and professional education. In scholarship reconsidered. In: Moser D, Todd R, Braxton J, Associates, editors. . San Francisco, CA: Jossey Bass; 2016. p. 31–9.

Beach A. Boyer's impact on faculty development. In: Moser D, Ream TC, Braxton JM, Associates, editors. Scholarship reconsidered: priorities of the professoriate. San Francisco, CA: Jossey-Bass; 2016. p. 13–8.. Expanded Edition.

Beattie D. Expanding the view of scholarship: introduction. Acad Med. 2000;75:871–6.

Beaulieu M, Breton M, Brousselle A. Conceptualising 20 years of engaged scholarship: a scoping review. PLoS One. 2018;13(2):e0193201. https://doi.org/10.1371/journal.pone.0193201.

Bereiter C, Scardamalia M. Surpassing ourselves. Chicago, IL; La Salle, IL: Open Court; 1993.

Blackmore P. Prestige in academic life: excellence and exclusion. Abingdon: Routledge; 2016.

Boyer E. Scholarship reconsidered: priorities of the professoriate. Carnegie Foundation for the Advancement of Teaching. Princeton, NJ: Princeton University Press; 1990.

Boyer E. The scholarship of engagement. J Publ Serv Outreach. 1996;1:11–20.

Braxton J. Reflections on a scholarship of practice. Rev High Educ. 2005;28:285–93.

Burrage J, Shattell M, Habermann B. The scholarship of engagement in nursing. Nurs Outlook. 2005;53:220–3.

Checkoway B. Strengthening the scholarship of engagement in higher education. J High Educ Outreach Engag. 2013;17:7–21.

Chinn P, Falk-Rafael A. Embracing the focus of the discipline of nursing: critical caring pedagogy. J Nurs Scholarsh. 2018;50:687–94.

Diers D. Clinical scholarship. Image. 1995;11:24–30.

Fung D. Strength-based scholarship and good education: the scholarship circle. Innov Educ Teach Int. 2017;54:101–10.

Glassick C, Huber M, Maeroff G. Scholarship assessed: evaluation of the professoriate. San Francisco, CA: Jossey-Bass; 1997.

Hall E. Scholars and scholarship. Scand J Caring Sci. 2001;15:273–4.

Huber M. Teaching travels: reflections on the social life of classroom inquiry and innovation. Int J Schol Teach Learn. 2009;3(2):2. https://doi.org/10.20429/ijsotl.2009.030202.

Hutchings P, Shulman L. The scholarship of teaching: new elaborations, new developments. Change. 1999;31:10–5.

Jacelon C, Donoghue L, Breslin E. Scholar in residence: an innovative application of the scholarship of engagement. J Prof Nurs. 2010;2:61–6.

Kreber C, Cranton P. Exploring the scholarship of teaching. J High Educ. 2000;71:476–95.

Kreber C. Teaching excellence, teaching expertise, and the scholarship of teaching. Innov High Educ. 2002;27:5–23.

Kreindler S, Dowd D, Star N, Gottschalk T. Silos and social identity: the social identity approach as a framework for understanding and overcoming divisions in healthcare. Milbank Q. 2012;90:347–74.

McDaniels M, Skogsberg E. The scholars we need: preparing transdisciplinary professionals by leveraging the scholarship of practice. In: Braxton J, editor. New directions for higher education. San Francisco, CA: Jossey Bass; 2017. p. 71–83.

Nash M. Transdisciplinary training: key components and prerequisites for success. Am J Prev Med. 2008;35:S133–40.

Nurse P. Ensuring a successful research endeavour. The Nurse Review of UK Research Councils, Department of Business Innovations and Skills (BIS/1/624). 2015. Accessed from https://www.gov.uk/government/uploads/system/uploads/attachment_data/file/478125/BIS-15-625-ensuring-a-successful-UK-research-endeavour.pdf.

Peterson K, Stevens J. Integrating the scholarship of practice into the nurse academician portfolio. J Nurs Educ Pract. 2013;3:84–92.

Pinar W. What is curriculum theory? 2nd ed. New York, NY: Routledge; 2012.

Schon D. Knowing-in-action: the new scholarship requires a new epistemology. Change. 1995;27:27–34.

Shulman L. Teaching as community property: putting an end to pedagogical solitude. Change. 1993;26:6–7.

Simpson R. Toward a scholarship of outreach and engagement in higher education. J High Educ Outreach Engag. 2000;6:7–12.

Starck P. Boyer's multidimensional nature of scholarship: a new framework for schools of nursing. J Prof Nurs. 1996;12:268–76.

Thompson D. Is nursing viable as an academic discipline? Nurse Educ Today. 2009;29:694–7.

Trigwell K, Martin E, Benjamin J, Prosser M. Scholarship of teaching: a model. High Educ Res Dev. 2000;19:155–68.

Trigwell K, Shale S. Student learning and the scholarship of university teaching. Stud High Educ. 2004;29:523–36.

Transforming Advanced Practice Nursing into Clinical Scholarship

3.1 Introduction

The basis for transforming scholarly practice into clinical scholarship is referred to as ground-breaking work and therefore should not be diluted in any way. The notion that clinical scholarship is elusive in nursing is explored. Standards are presented that provide a platform to adjudicate scholarly work across the dimensions of scholarship. A scholarship of practice is outlined and opens a dialogue in the context of advanced practice nursing. Scholarship in nursing is considered in light of Boyer's seminal work when he considered scholarship in the context of practice disciplines, in particular, in schools, communities, and universities. In this framework Boyer proposed domains of scholarship which go beyond research and publication and can be seen to work separately or interdependently (Boyer 1990). According to the AACN (1999) the scholarship of application (practice) is where the emphasis is placed on the use of new knowledge in solving society's problems. Further, essential standards to adjudicate on scholarly work provide a framework for the uniform evaluation of clinical scholarship.

3.2 Pillars of Scholarship and Clinical Scholarship

There is a growing acceptance that knowledge from various sources is required to solve the complex challenges that arise in clinical practice. The strategies used for knowledge production have also expanded to include various approaches beyond pure research and are described by Boyer (1990) as four overlapping, yet interdependent domains; discovery, integration, application and teaching. The scholarship of discovery, traditionally viewed as 'research', results in the generation of new knowledge or support for existing knowledge; the scholarship of integration refers to the connectedness of known knowledge to new interpretations; the scholarship of teaching includes the study of how students learn and the exploration of teaching strategies, and the scholarship of application is the application of knowledge outside the academic setting to the wider community.

© Springer Nature Switzerland AG 2019
L. O'Connor, *The Nature of Scholarship, a Career Legacy Map and Advanced Practice*, Advanced Practice in Nursing, https://doi.org/10.1007/978-3-319-91695-8_3

Boyer's view of the scholarship of application is principally pertinent to the practice professions, where understanding is generated through the application of knowledge to solve problems in clinical areas, or anywhere where nursing is practiced. Furthermore, supporting all nurses in clinical practice to produce knowledge can strengthen nursing's capacity to generate meaningful knowledge for practice and the profession. Moreover, a clear understanding of clinical scholarship will continue to assist in the development of the next generation of nurse scholars.

Clinical nursing scholarship is viewed as necessary to advance nursing knowledge and through this knowledge, contribute to improved health services and patient care (Diers 1995; Schlotfeldt 1992). Later, the use of Boyer's framework was used to promote scholarship (Starck 1996), to appreciate that scholarship is broader than traditional research and to encourage schools of nursing to establish policies to support this expanded view of scholarship. However, more recent discussions of clinical scholarship in relation to Boyer's (1990) framework are sparse. Understanding clinical scholarship in Boyer's framework can generate dialogue and increase the precision of knowledge derived from practice, and in particular for the advanced practice nursing practitioner/aspirant in the context of explicating their scholarly activities.

The scholarly literature was searched from 1983 to 2015 by Limoges and Acorn (2016) to explicate clinical scholarship as being synonymous with the scholarship of application and to explore the evolution of scholarly practice to clinical scholarship. They used Boyer's scholarship of application to draw analytical conclusions. Boyer (1990) described the scholarship of application as applying knowledge in community or service activities, with the outcomes of benefit to the larger community. Accordingly, clinical scholarship was defined as the scholarship of application conducted by clinicians (Limoges and Acorn 2016, p. 749). Furthermore, the approaches to knowledge production for clinical scholarship and the scholarship of application were found to be linked and involve systematic observation, synthesis, application of knowledge and dissemination (Limoges et al. 2015; Wilkes et al. 2013; Grigsby and Thorndyke 2011). Both involve relaying the knowledge produced in ways that include the rationale and the elements of practice that generated the outcomes (Grigsby and Thorndyke 2011). Documenting and disseminating knowledge produced to make it available for critique is an important feature, not just to align with the criteria of scholarship, but also so that it can be used, reused, shared and built on (Limoges and Acorn 2016). Therefore, drawing parallels between clinical scholarship and the scholarship of application can bring recognition to clinical scholarship by aligning it with Boyer's (1990) well known knowledge framework. Clinical scholarship requires expert clinical knowledge, creativity, knowledge of research, interpersonal skills and evidence-based practices, while supporting the development of best practice standards and the dissemination of nursing knowledge (Wilkes et al. 2013).

For a clear understanding of clinical scholarship and how to support its development within advanced practice nursing, a discussion is warranted on the differences between 'scholarly nursing practice' and 'clinical scholarship'. Scholarly nursing practice requires an astute interpretation of research to achieve currency in best practices, evidence based practice (EBP), monitoring of care outcomes and continuous inquiry to improve nursing care to achieve favourable outcomes. Characteristics such as confidence, being available to others to share expertise and being an active learner, are associated with scholarly practice (Riley and Beal 2013). This level of practice is conducted with a sense of ownership, creativity, autonomy (STTI 1999), passion and vision (Riley and Beal 2013; Wilkes et al. 2013). Advanced practice nursing practitioners engaged in scholarly nursing practice are ideally situated to identify areas requiring additional knowledge or understanding paving the way for a quality patient care sustained agenda enactment in the practice setting. However, their work needs to meet the criteria of critical reflectivity, scrutiny by peers and an ethic of inquiry (Andresen 2000) to be considered as scholarship.

By aligning projects to Boyer's framework from the conception of an idea through to implementation and dissemination, nurses can structure their projects to ensure that they meet the recognised criteria for scholarship. Using this understanding can also guide them to recognise where they may require assistance and seek it to ensure success (Limoges and Acorn 2016, p. 750). An important first step to promote the transitions of scholarly nursing practice to clinical scholarship is to identify nurses engaged in scholarly practice (clinical scholars) and the clinical leaders in a setting. Nurses exhibiting scholarly practice become 'clinical leaders' when they share their expertise and guide other nurses to improve clinical practice (Limoges and Acorn 2016, p. 750). Accordingly, the knowledge generated through such scholarly nursing practice can be developed into clinical scholarship (Rocco et al. 2015; Riley and Beal 2013; Riley et al. 2007). Support is necessary for clinical nurses to have their work documented, peer reviewed and disseminated (Limoges and Acorn 2016, p. 750). Moreover, nursing care that achieves positive outcomes to nurse sensitive quality indicators or gaps identified through quality assurance initiatives are agenda topics for clinical scholarship (Rocco et al. 2015; Tymkow 2014).

3.2.1   Clinical Scholarship Is Elusive in Nursing

The way the word and concept of "scholarship" is used in nursing reflects ambiguity and inconsistency. For the most part scholarship is considered unidimensional (Starck 1996, p. 268). Scholarship is also elusive, like quality; it is known when seen, but it is hard to define; only a scholar can recognise scholarship. Moreover, "scholarship is associated with high standards of excellence, rigorous science, and attention to detail as well as thoroughness and comprehensiveness" (Starck 1996, p. 268).

According to Maeve (1994) the scholarship of the bedside nurse, or bedside scholar, is one in which the worth of that scholarship is made visible and tangible to patients, to other nurses, and to society as a whole. A mosaicism of nursing scholarship is an exciting prospect that affords opportunities for all nurses, not just those involved in research and publication, to disseminate the language of their stories that captures the knowledge, meanings, and essences of their practice, just as their pens can delineate the pathway through the swamp as they tell their stories (Maeve 1994). In doing so, nurses engage in the process of constructing and reconstructing practice (Street 1990). It is vital that nurses all enter into the dialogue of scholarship and knowledge development in nursing; for we are diminished by the voices we do not hear (Maeve 1994). Advanced practice nursing practitioners/aspirants are ideally located to ensure that nursing practice is conceptualised as scholarly and each of the domains of Boyer's scholarship can be used as a precursor to entering that dialogue of scholarship, thereby making visible the full potential of their contributions to health and health care.

In the context of contemporary nursing the crucial need for clinical leadership and clinical expertise abounds. In conjunction with this there was a cry for clinical scholarship in the late 1990s and Sigma Theta Tau International (STTI 1999) espoused that clinical scholarship was "an approach which enables evidence-based nursing and the development of best practice to meet the needs of clients efficiently and effectively" (p. 4). This influential international society goes on to state that clinical scholarship can only flourish if both clinical and academic organisations embrace it (Mannix et al. 2013). If scholarship is at the heart of what a profession is, then clinical scholarship must be central to the nursing discipline (Boyer 1990). The discipline's philosophy, theory and practice are intertwined and as reflected in Boyer's ideas; scholarship in nursing can come from four scholarly activities: discovery, integration, application, and teaching. It is argued by Starck (1996) that clinical scholarship, while having significant focus on practice, would also bridge the other three scholarly activities. According to Roger's (1966) seminal work, "nursing's future as a learned profession and its potential for human service is dependent on the extent to which scholarly education through doctoral study in nursing is made explicit" (p. 75). Furthermore, Kitson (2006) stated emphatically, that "true scholarship is both the breadth and depth of knowledge an individual has in a particular subject area" (p. 540) and its development is essential to the nursing discipline, and doctorates grounded in clinical practice will build a stronger culture of inquiry and scholarship in the clinical environment. Nursing needs scholars and nursing provides a service to society which, in the majority of developed countries, accounts for the largest recurrent expenditure that has to be built upon sound knowledge, theories, principles, methods and practices. Of note, 20 years ago, Kitson (1999) advocated, it is now the time that metaphorical scaffolding was erected around the edifice of knowledge generation in nursing: and not before time, which still holds relevancy for today.

Mannix et al. (2013) sought to determine clinical nurses' understandings of clinical scholarship with an emphasis on clinicians' perceptions of the differences in the construct of the roles of clinical scholar, clinical expert and clinical leader (Mannix et al. 2013). 18 nurses employed in a clinical role and who were students (Master of Nursing or Doctorates) were recruited through a modified snowballing approach at five universities (one in Canada, three in England and one in Australia) (Mannix et al. 2013). While the emphasis of this project was defining clinical scholarship, it became apparent that the nurse participants saw distinct differences in being a clinical scholar, clinical expert or clinical leader. The ideal for the majority of participants was for a nurse to be a combination of clinical scholar and clinical leader or clinical scholar with clinical expertise or a combination of all three. The nurse participants felt scholarship was particularly important for a clinical expert (Mannix et al. 2013). The clinical experts were seen to translate research outcomes into local practice, viewed as doing research projects but often not disseminating this to the broader community. For some nurses, there was a perception that clinical scholarship and expertise were different but there was some uncertainty about the exact nature of the differences (Mannix et al. 2013).

The clinical scholar was considered to be more academically focused in gaining their knowledge base, while still drawing on the knowledge gained from their own clinical experience. Mannix et al. (2013) illustrated that one participant identified a clinical scholar as a person who is able to disseminate *to a very broad audience and to be peer reviewed on what you write or speak and it's like scholarship cannot take place by you, it has to be in the broader nursing community.* The findings reflect the curiosity of the clinical scholar; the linking of theory and practice by doing practice-based research, the development of an environment to share the results of research with a broader community, and the nature and impact of nursing. Motivation and inspiration were also found to be important aspects of the role of the clinical scholar (Mannix et al. 2013).

The qualities of a scholar are identified in the literature embedded in the dimensions of scholarship articulated by Boyer which is consistently relevant to the debate regarding clinical scholarship and advanced practice nursing practitioners. The qualities are linked with Glassick et al.'s work (1997) and also Andresen (2000) that relate to scholarly knowing; scrutiny by peers, public and self (see Fig. 4.1, Chap. 4). Certain qualities associated with a scholar's character are recognised by virtually all higher education institutions as consequential not only for the individual professor but for the entire community of scholars (Glassick et al. 1997, p. 61). In considering the qualities of a scholar three characteristics merit especial consideration: *integrity, perseverance* and *courage* and should serve as a reminder that scholarship has a moral aspect that should feature in all its dimensions: discovery, teaching, integration, and application (Glassick et al. 1997, pp. 63–67).

The move to broaden scholarship called new attention to the imperative for improved standards that allow colleagues, peers, and other scholars make reliable judgements about quality without overreliance on quantification. It is generally recognised that new means of evaluation are essential to foster first rate research and creative work and to encourage and reward scholarly teaching and professional service (Glassick et al. 1997, p. 20).

3.2.2   Essential Standards to Adjudicate on Scholarly Work

Following Boyer, Glassick et al. (1997) focused on evaluating the work of scholars. Their six standards of scholarly activity for review are: clear goals; adequate preparation; appropriate methods; significant results; effective presentation and reflective critique. One outstanding characteristic critical to the assessment of all areas of scholarship is the importance of presentation to others. Discovery of new knowledge or integration of previously published information into a novel synthesis does not contribute to scholarship unless it is communicated to others. Experimental results from scientific experiments that remain forever in a lab notebook have no intrinsic value (Beattie 2000, p. 874). To be considered scholarship, every scholarly accomplishment needs to be shared with and judged by other scholars (Huber 2016). Each standard is pertinent to making visible the work of the advanced practice nursing practitioner, and especially highlighted in the purpose of scholarship illustrated in the category of 'effective presentation':

Scholarship, however brilliant, lacks fulfilment without someone on the receiving end. The discovery should be made known to more than the discoverer; teaching is not teaching without students; integration makes scant contribution unless it is communicated so that people can benefit from it; and application becomes application by addressing others' needs (Glassick et al. 1997, p. 31). The aforementioned authors query whether scholars are using 'appropriate forums' for their intended audiences: 'Does the scholar present his or her message with clarity and integrity?' (p. 32). They state that as 'a public act', which needs 'a sense of audience', scholarship benefits from using new technologies and media. Certainly, more than presentation, it requires the capability to listen to and interact with one's audiences:

Effective presentation … may require the scholar to do more listening than speaking, recognising that what the audience says is part of communication (Glassick et al. 1997, p. 32). There is an important emphasis here on the principle of multi-way communication, which enables scholars to engage productively with different communities and cultures, whether academic, professional or public (Fung 2017).

Furthermore, Glassick et al. (1997) identified that their set of six standards be widely used across disciplines to evaluate basic research, applied work, interdisciplinary projects, and teaching. Together, these standards map a common arc of intellectual endeavour. With appropriate adjustments Huber (2016) argued that these six standards could be applied well to the four kinds of scholarship identified in *Scholarship Reconsidered* and provide a framework for uniformity in the evaluation of scholarship (p. xiii). Whatever the scholarly emphasis, the approach deserves dignity and respect, insofar as it is performed with distinction. Accordingly, excellence must be the only yardstick (Glassick et al. 1997).

Clearly, evaluation that uses different standards for research, teaching, and professional service has outlived its day (Glassick et al. 1997, p. 23). The paradox is this: in order to recognise discovery, integration, application, and teaching as legitimate forms of scholarship, the academy must evaluate them by a set of standards that capture and acknowledge what they share as scholarly acts (Glassick et al. 1997). All works of scholarship, be they discovery, integration, application, or teaching, involve a continuous sequence of unfolding stages and when people praise a work of scholarship, they usually mean that the project in question shows that it has been guided by these six qualitative standards (p. 24):

1. Clear goals
2. Adequate preparation
3. Appropriate methods
4. Significant results
5. Effective presentation
6. Reflective critique

According to Glassick et al. (1997) there is a common language in which to discuss the standards for scholarly work of all kinds, a language that enables scholars and assessors to see clearly what discovery, integration, application, and teaching share as scholarly activities. They acknowledge that the six standards define phases of an intellectual process that are in reality not so neatly categorised (Glassick et al. 1997). The questions directed towards each of the six standards (see Fig. 3.1) could become a significant prompt for the advanced practice nursing practitioner/aspirant throughout the design of their career legacy portfolio and in particular during the iterative phases of creating their career legacy map (see Chap. 6) that hones in on their scholarly activities.

Clear goals

Does the scholar state the basic purposes of his or her work clearly?

Does the scholar define objectives that are realistic and achievable?

Does the scholar identify important questions in the field?

Adequate preparation

Does the scholar show an understanding of existing scholarship in the field?

Does the scholar bring the necessary skills to his or her work?

Does the scholar bring together the resources necessary to move the project forward?

Appropriate methods

Does the scholar use methods appropriate to the goals?

Does the scholar apply effectively the methods selected?

Does the scholar modify procedures in response to changing circumstances?

Significant results

Does the scholar achieve the goals?

Does the scholar's work add consequentially to the field?

Does the scholar's work open additional areas for further exploration?

Effective presentation

Does the scholar use a suitable style and effective organisation to present his or her work?

Does the scholar use appropriate forums for communicating work to its intended audience?

Does the scholar present his or her message with clarity and integrity?

Reflective critique

Does the scholar critically evaluate his or her own work?

Does the scholar bring an appropriate breadth of evidence to his or her critique?

Does the scholar use evaluation to improve the quality of future work?
(Glassick et al. 1997, p.36).

Source: C.E. Glassick, M.T. Huber, and G.I. Maeroff. 1997. Scholarship Assessed: Evaluation of the Professoriate. San Francisco, Jossey-Bass.

Fig. 3.1 Summary of standards

3.3   Scholarship of Practice

Scholarship is, in a way, an invitation—a challenge—to reconsider our identity as language educators: it suggest an identity that expands into areas often occluded in the past to one that is more visible, more vocal, making contributions to professional knowledge, exerting influence, shaping practices and policies, engaging with students differently and accumulating social and epistemic capital and recognition (Ding 2016, p. 13).

The impact of Boyer's work on the disciplines is evident in how scholarship is being applied to improve disciplinary practice. According to Kielhofner (2005a) there is evidence of Boyer's impact in the development of a "scholarship of practice", which seeks to bridge the gap between theories developed and research findings obtained by academicians and the questions asked and approaches adopted by practitioners in their daily work. Practitioners assert that theory and research are often irrelevant to their everyday work and difficult to implement due to the tendency for academicians to emphasize scientific rigor over relevance (Kielhofner 2005a). The scholarship of practice addresses the concern about the relevance and utility for practice (e.g., ease, efficiency, and effectiveness of professional communication) and graduate education of the theories developed and research findings obtained by academicians (Kielhofner 2005b). By coupling knowledge generation and knowledge use "into a single enterprise", the scholarship of practice recognizes that there is knowledge in practice in addition to knowledge for practice (Kielhofner 2005b).

Pursuit of that scholarship of practice improves practice in both soft- and hard-applied disciplines, while Biglan (1973a, b) characterized academic disciplines as having pure-applied as well as hard-soft dimensions. Soft disciplines (e.g., nursing, occupational therapy, business and accounting) have lower levels of paradigmatic development (Lyken-Segosebe 2017). Practitioners in these disciplines exhibit less agreement regarding appropriate research questions for their field and appropriate methodologies for addressing these questions, while, hard disciplines (e.g., pharmacy, engineering and agriculture) have high paradigmatic development (Lyken-Segosebe 2017, p. 22). That said, specifically, Boyer asserts that in conducting scholarship of application, the scholar addresses the question: "How can knowledge be responsibly applied to consequential problems? How can it be helpful to individuals as well as institutions?" And further, "Can social problems themselves define an agenda for scholarly investigation"? (Boyer 1990, p. 21). Moreover, these questions posed by Boyer should be part of the repertoire of advanced practice nursing practitioners' scholarly practice agenda.

Indeed, some nurse academicians function as advanced practice nursing practitioners who engage in clinical practice activities while advancing their scholarly agenda. In addition to their traditional scholarly roles as faculty members, advanced practice nursing practitioners have added responsibilities (e.g., legal responsibilities for safe practice) and must satisfy the professional standards (e.g., certification and competency requirements) associated with clinical practice within the discipline (Peterson and Stevens 2013). This dual role of nurse-academic and nurse-clinician has led to practice being specifically recognized as part of scholarship by the American Association of Colleges of Nursing (AACN). The AACN formally recognized the scholarship of practice as a form of knowledge generation. In its position paper 20 years ago, *Defining Scholarship for the Discipline of Nursing*, the AACN (1999) defines scholarship pursued by academic-tenure-track or clinical-track nursing faculty as:

> *those activities that systematically advance the teaching, research and practice of nursing through rigorous inquiry that (1) is significant to the profession, (2) is creative, (3) can be documented, (4) can be replicated or elaborated, and (5) can be peer-reviewed through various methods (p. 2).*

Within nursing, the scholarship of practice applies nursing and related knowledge to the assessment and validation of patient care outcomes, the measurement of quality-of-life indicators, the development and refinement of practice protocols/strategies, the evaluation of systems of care, and the analysis of innovative health care delivery models (AACN 1999). Research findings from the scholarship of practice are directly applied in procedures, clinical protocols, and practice guidelines (Riley et al. 2002). One of the basic principles of a scholarship of practice is the changed role of the investigator from expert to collaborator and facilitator who engages the target population or sample-the client or patient-in a cooperative partnership relationship and with appropriate sensitivity (Burgener 2001). Nursing practice models, especially in advanced practice nursing, bring essential expertise to the health care arena that addresses both quality and access problems. Clinical scholarship activities are an important vehicle for studying and articulating these skills. Therefore, the data derived from these scholarly activities are needed to describe nursing's commitment to patients and to highlight the particular ability of nurses to address the complex needs of people and systems (Fiand et al. 2004).

The scholarship of application, or *practice scholarship*, encompasses all aspects of the delivery of nursing services. Competence in practice is the method by which *knowledge in the profession* is both advanced and applied. Components of the scholarship of practice includes the development of clinical knowledge which entails systematic development and application of theoretical formulations and the conduct of clinically applicable research and evaluation studies in clinical areas of expertise (AACN 1999). Cameron-Traub (1995) considered scholarship in nursing to include three activities: conceptual processes (rationality; thinking), clinical processes (through practice) and empirical processes (through sensory perception). That said, the effort to broaden the meaning of scholarship simply cannot succeed until the academy has clear standards for evaluating this wider range of scholarly work (Glassick et al. 1997, p. 5).

Eighteen years ago, Burgener (2001) stated very concisely, "foremost among those expected outcomes of the scholarship of practice is that more use of practice-based research methods will contribute to the goal of finding answers to real-world health problems" (p. 53). An individual's potential for performance in any role is enormous, especially if it is not restricted and constrained from the onset. Therefore, it is time to view faculty practice with a wider vision, to allow the full development of each individual person as a true scholar (Newland and Truglio-Londrigan 2003, p. 277). In these faculty practice partnerships, nursing faculty have access to subjects for their research and clinicians have access to research experts and consultation. The outcomes of such partnerships include enhanced evidence-based practice, increased grant funding, and overall improvement in the "generation, dissemination, and application of knowledge for the improvement of nursing practice and patient outcomes" (Dreher et al. 2001, p. 114). As far back as 2007, based on Boyer's definition of scholarship, the following definition of faculty practice was recommended: "Faculty practice is the provision of direct and indirect nursing care with the goal of integrating the four missions of the School of Nursing: scholarship, professional practice, teaching, and service. Direct modalities include interventions or services for individuals, families, groups, communities, and systems, while indirect modalities include education, mentoring, leadership, collaboration, consultation and research" (Becker et al. 2007, p. 51). According to Newland and Truglio-Londrigan (2003) the question that warrants an answer is how can faculty practice be integrated within the institution's cultural values? Practice has never left nursing education but has become an optional add-on rather than an integral component of the traditional academic triad model; hence the structure of faculty roles within nursing education must facilitate faculty practice to ensure this reconnection (Newland and Truglio-Londrigan 2003, p. 277). A survey was mailed to the membership of the National Organisation of Nurse Practitioner Faculties to examine the differences between practicing faculty who were tenured and those who were non-tenured and to identify predictors of tenure in the USA with a 50% response (n = 452) obtained (Pohl et al. 2012). The findings revealed that more than three quarters of the sample (76%, n = 343) were practicing, and another 20% (n = 91) indicated that although they were not practicing, others at their institutions were engaged in clinical practice. Another 4% (n = 18) reported that no faculty members were practicing at their institutions. Of note, more than 51% reported that practice was not considered in either promotion or tenure decisions at their institution (Pohl et al. 2012). However, more than half (55%) of the respondents reported that faculty practice at their institution integrated practice, teaching, and research. This highlights a conflict for practicing faculty. If practice is encouraged or required, it needs to be recognised in promotion and tenure when there are scholarly outcomes (Pohl et al. 2012).

The challenge currently is for nursing faculty to ensure that the integration of practitioner, educator and researcher roles are explicit rather than elusive across the dimensions of discovery, integration, application, teaching and engagement. The debate warrants further exploration as the scholarship of practice would require specific and consistent resources to enact its essence such as outreach scholarship as a community process. The interesting scenario here is that advanced practice nursing practitioners are ideally placed to participate in the scholarship of application via faculty practice partnerships on account of their access to service users and key stakeholders aligned with their local, national and international health policy context agenda.

3.4 Conclusion

Clinical nursing scholarship was viewed as necessary to advance nursing knowledge. Understanding clinical scholarship in Boyer's framework can generate dialogue and increase the precision of knowledge derived from practice. For a clear understanding of clinical scholarship and how to support its development, a discussion is warranted on the differences between 'scholarly nursing practice' and 'clinical scholarship'. Scholarly nursing practice requires an astute interpretation of research to achieve currency in best practices, evidence based practice (EBP), monitoring of care outcomes and continuous inquiry to improve nursing care to achieve favourable health outcomes.

Advanced practice nursing practitioners engaged in scholarly practice are ideally situated to identify areas requiring additional knowledge or understanding for enactment of a quality patient-centered agenda. However, their work needs to meet the criteria of critical reflectivity, scrutiny by peers and an ethic of inquiry (Andresen 2000) to be considered as scholarship. By aligning projects to Boyer's framework from the conception of the idea through to implementation and dissemination, projects can be structured to ensure that they meet the recognised criteria for scholarship.

Advanced practice nursing practitioners are ideally located to ensure that nursing practice is conceptualised as scholarly and each of the domains of Boyer's scholarship can be used as a precursor to entering that dialogue of clinical scholarship thereby making visible the full potential of their contributions to health and their role in shaping health care delivery. If scholarship is at the heart of what a profession is, then clinical scholarship must be central to the nursing discipline (Boyer 1990).

Six standards were identified that map a common arc of intellectual endeavour: clear goals, adequate preparation, appropriate methods, significant results, effective presentation, and reflective critique (Glassick et al. 1997). With appropriate adjustments Huber (2016) argued that these standards could be applied well to the four domains of scholarship identified in *Scholarship Reconsidered* and provide a framework for uniformity in the evaluation of scholarship (p. xiii). One outstanding characteristic critical to the assessment of all areas of scholarship is the importance of presentation to others. To be considered scholarship, every scholarly accomplishment needs to be shared with and judged by other scholars (Huber 2016). Whatever the scholarly emphasis, the approach deserves dignity and respect, insofar as it is performed with distinction. Excellence must be the only yardstick (Glassick et al. 1997).

Within nursing, the scholarship of practice applies nursing and related knowledge to the assessment and validation of patient care outcomes, the measurement of quality-of-life indicators, the construction and transformation of practice protocols/strategies, the evaluation of systems of care, and the critical analysis of innovative health care delivery models. Research findings from the scholarship of practice are then directly applied in interventions, clinical protocols, and evidence-based practice guidelines.

Faculty practice was defined and there was a consensus presented that the question no longer is whether nursing faculty practice is essential but rather how can that faculty practice be integrated within the institution's cultural values. This was identified as important because practice is perceived as an optional add-on rather than an integral component of the traditional academic triad model of research, teaching and service.

References

American Association of Colleges of Nursing. Position statement on defining scholarship for the discipline of nursing. 1999. Accessed from http://www.aacn.nche.edu/publications/position/defining-scholarship.

Andresen L. A useable, trans-disciplinary conception of scholarship. High Educ Res Dev. 2000;19:137–53.

Beattie D. Expanding the view of scholarship. Acad Med. 2000;75:871–5.

Becker K, Dang D, Jordan E, Kub J, Welch A, Smith C, White K. An evaluation framework for faculty practice. Nurs Outlook. 2007;55:44–54.

Biglan A. The characteristics of subject matter in different academic areas. J Appl Psychol. 1973a;57:195–203.

Biglan A. Relationships between subject matter characteristics and the structure and output of university departments. J Appl Psychol. 1973b;57:204–13.

Boyer E. Scholarship reconsidered: priorities of the professoriate. San Francisco, CA: Jossey-Bass; 1990.

Burgener S. Scholarship of practice for a practice profession. J Prof Nurs. 2001;17:46–54.

Cameron-Traub E. Clinical, conceptual and empirical aspects of nursing practice. In: Gray G, Pratt R, editors. Scholarship in the discipline of nursing. Melbourne, VIC: Churchill Livingstone; 1995. p. 1–20.

Diers D. Clinical scholarship. Image. 1995;11:28–30.

Ding A. Challenging scholarship: a thought piece. Language Scholar. 2016. Accessed from http://languagescholar.leeds.ac.uk/. ISSN:2398-8509.

Dreher M, Everett L, Hartwig S. The University of Iowa nursing collaboratory: a partnership for creative education and practice. J Prof Nurs. 2001;17:114–20.

Fiand TK, Barr K, Hille G, Pelish P, Pozehl B, Hulme P, Muhlbauer S, Burge S. Identifying clinical scholarship guidelines for faculty practice. J Prof Nurs. 2004;20:147–55.

Fung D. Strength-based scholarship and good education: the scholarship circle. Innov Educ Teach Int. 2017;54:101–10.

Grigsby R, Thorndyke L. Perspective: recognising and rewarding clinical scholarship. Acad Med. 2011;86:127–31.

Glassick C, Huber M, Maeroff G. Scholarship assessed: evaluation of the professoriate. San Francisco: Jossey-Bass; 1997.

Huber, T. (2016) Foreword. In Moser D, Ream TC, Braxton JM, and Associates Scholarship reconsidered: priorities of the professoriate, San Francisco, CA. Jossey-Bass. Expanded Edition..

Kielhofner G. A scholarship of practice: creating discourse between theory, research and practice. In: Crist P, Kielhofner G, editors. The scholarship of practice: academic practice collaborations for promoting occupational therapy. New York, NY: Haworth Press; 2005a. p. 7–16.

Kielhofner G. Research concepts in clinical scholarship---scholarship and practice: bridging the divide. Am J Occup Ther. 2005b;59:231–9.

Kitson A. The relevance of scholarship for nursing research and practice. J Adv Nurs. 1999;29:773–5.

Kitson A. The relevance of scholarship for nursing research and practice. J Adv Nurs. 2006;55:541–3.

Lyken-Segosebe D. The scholarship of practice. Appl Discip. 2017;178:21–33.

Limoges J, Acorn S. Transforming practice into clinical scholarship. J Adv Nurs. 2016;72:747–53.

Limoges J, Acorn S, Osborne M. The scholarship of application: recognising and promoting nurses contribution to knowledge development. J Contin Educ Nurs. 2015;46:77–82.

Maeve M. The carrier bag theory of nursing practice. Adv Nurs Sci. 1994;16:9–22.

Mannix J, Wilkes L, Jackson D. Marking out the clinical expert/clinical leader/clinical scholar: perspectives from nurses in the clinical area. BMC Nurs. 2013;12:12.. Accessed from https://bmcnurs.biomedcentral.com/articles/10.1186/1472-6955-12-12

Newland J, Truglio-Londrigan M. Faculty practice: facilitation of clinical integrations into the academic triad model. J Prof Nurs. 2003;19:269–78.

Peterson K, Stevens J. Integrating the scholarship of practice into the nurse academician portfolio. J Nurs Educ Pract. 2013;3:84–92.

Pohl J, Duderstadt K, Tolve-Schoeneberger C, Uphold C, Hartig M. Faculty practice: what do the data show? Findings from the NONPF faculty practice survey. Nurs Outlook. 2012;60:250–8.

Riley J, Beal J, Levi P, McCausland M. Revisioning nursing scholarship. J Nurs Scholarsh. 2002;34:383–9.

Riley J, Beal J, Lancaster D. Scholarly nursing practice from the perspectives of experienced nurses. J Adv Nurs. 2007;61:425–35.

Riley J, Beal J. Scholarly nursing practice from the perspectives of early-career nurses. Nurs Outlook. 2013;61:E16–24.

Rogers C. On becoming a person. London: Constable; 1966.

Rocco G, Affonso D, Mayberry L, Sasso L, Stievano A, Alvaro R. Center of excellence to build nursing scholarship and improve health care in Italy. J Nurs Scholarsh. 2015;47:170–7.

Schlotfeldt R. Why promote clinical nursing scholarship? Clin Nurs Res. 1992;1:5–8.

Starck P. Boyer's multidimensional nature of scholarship: a new framework for schools of nursing. J Prof Nurs. 1996;12:268–76.

Street A. A nursing practice-high, hard ground, messy swamps and the pathways in between. Burwood, VIC: Deakin; 1990.

STTI. Sigma Theta Tau International Clinical Scholarship resource paper. 1999. Accessed on 17 December 2018, from http://www.nursingsociety.org/about-stti/position-statements-and-resource-papers.

Tymkow C. Clinical scholarship and evidence-based practice. In: Zaccagnini M, White K, editors. The doctor of nursing practice essentials: a new model for advanced practice nursing. 2nd ed. Sudbury, MA: Jones and Barlett; 2014. p. 62–9.

Wilkes L, Mannix J, Jackson D. Practicing nurses perspectives of clinical scholarship: a qualitative study. BMC Nurs. 2013;12:21–7.

The Spectrum of Clinical Scholarship

4

4.1 Introduction

The spectrum of clinical scholarship is designed in the context of the advanced practice nursing practitioner across the interdependent dimensions of the scholarship of engagement, integration, application, discovery and teaching and their respective indicators. Three characteristics associated with scholarship are illustrated and their elements that influence the scholarly activities of the advanced practice nursing practitioner are collectively explored as a platform to perfect their craft of inquiry within a landscape of clinical scholarship. Patient-centered care definitions and dimensions are described in depth and how nursing is constructed in the language of person-centered care is presented. The role of communities of practice is examined in light of their support for a culture of clinical scholarship and person-centered care that requires a sea-change in the mind-set of the practitioner and the recipient of the service.

4.2 Clinical Scholarship

Clinical Scholarship exists along a continuum of evidence-based practice, quality improvement and research. Nurses' active involvement in scholarly activities within a landscape of clinical scholarship is necessary to advance the nursing profession and improve patient outcomes. There is a lack of clarity about the various terms used to refer to scholarly activities-is it translational research, research use, implementation science, evidence-based practice (EBP), quality assurance, quality improvement (QI), or some combination of these? (Carter et al. 2017, p. 266).

Clinical nursing scholarship has been comprehensively defined as the following:

an approach that enables evidence-based nursing and development of best practices to meet the needs of clients efficiently and effectively. It requires the identification of desired outcomes; the use of systematic observation and scientifically-based methods to identify

© Springer Nature Switzerland AG 2019   45
L. O'Connor, *The Nature of Scholarship, a Career Legacy Map and Advanced Practice*, Advanced Practice in Nursing, https://doi.org/10.1007/978-3-319-91695-8_4

and solve clinical problems; the substantiation of practice and clinical decisions with refer-ence to scientific principles, current research, consensus-based guidelines, quality improve-ment data and other forms of evidence; the evaluation, documentation, and dissemination of outcomes and improvements in practice…and the use of clinical knowledge and expertise to anticipate trends, predict needs, create effective clinical products and services, and man-age outcomes (STTI 1999, p. 4).

Hence, clinical scholarship refers to nurses' active participation in activities that improve patient care, advance the nursing profession, and contribute to and build on new knowledge. Although evidence-based practice, quality improvement, and research are activities along the spectrum of clinical scholarship, recent studies have stressed the differences rather than similarities among them. The emphasis on such differences has promulgated the illusion that these activities are independent, creat-ing a rift rather than collaboration (Carter et al. 2017, p. 267).

In an attempt to arrive at more definitional clarity, STTI personified clinical nurs-ing scholarship via a description of clinical scholars; nurses who are curious, critical thinkers, reflectors on practice, who develop an environment of sharing the results of their research with the broader nursing and general community to improve effective-ness of clinical interventions (STTI 1999, p. 5). Certain qualities associated with a scholar's character are recognised by virtually all higher education institutions as consequential not only for the individual professor but for the entire community of scholars (Glassick et al. 1997, p. 61). In considering the qualities of a scholar, Glassick et al. (1997), propose that three characteristics merit especial consideration: *integrity, perseverance* and *courage*. To recognise these traits requires qualitative judgement, but this judgement need not be arbitrary when guided by a careful and impartial examination of the candidate (Glassick et al. 1997). The foundation of aca-demic life is based on integrity. In fact, scholarship cannot prosper without an atmo-sphere of trust. Therefore, at the most basic level, scholars must be truthful in reporting what they have done and their findings. The credibility of scholarly inquiry requires integrity so that those whose words and ideas the scholar has used receive appropriate credit (Glassick et al. 1997, p. 63). Scholars must gain confidence that through their courage to move beyond the ordinary they can enrich and further theo-retical knowledge, strengthen practical applications of knowledge, and demonstrate new ways of looking at the connecting points where different kinds of knowledge converge and persevere to perfect their craft (Glassick et al. 1997, p. 66). These qualities of character should serve as reminders that good scholarship involves more than doing one's job well, as important as that is, and such reminders should hold value for the advanced practice nursing practitioner/aspirant as they go about their day-to-day scholarly activities. Accordingly, Glassick et al. (1997) put forward six standards (see Chap. 3) to be embedded within the repertoire of the scholar so that evaluation and all activities connected to scholarship, including faculty development, self-evaluation and self-enrichment, have an ethical dimension (Glassick et al. 1997).

Clinical scholarship has an essential element of passion which will not only help nurses to challenge authority but motivate others to pursue scholarly activities (Wilkies et al. 2013). Consequently, Wilkies et al. (2013) sought to elucidate under-standings and develop a contextual definition of clinical scholarship for clinical nursing, using an interpretative approach with 18 practicing nurses from Australia,

Canada and England. Vision and passion were seen to be essential elements of all components of clinical scholarship. Through this vision and passion a clinical scholar *must be able to challenge, shift and rewrite clinical practice and not only do it in practice but in the academic world.* Therefore, as argued by the participants, clinical scholarship is easier for a nurse who has both a clinical, academic/research role. Clinical scholarship is exemplified in one participant's description of a clinical scholar: *a clinical nurse who is able to bring together many different knowledge bases which would include research, academia, evidence and practice disciplines in practice* (Wilkies et al. 2013, p. 4).

The keystone component of clinical scholarship for all the participants was that knowledge gained by any scholarly endeavour must be made public as described; *scholarship is a continuum from clinical practice to publication ... been a driver for change in nursing practice* (Wilkies et al. 2013, p. 5). Therefore, clinical scholarship involves identifying issues in practice and beginning *to explore how we can address the uncertainties that we face in practice today* (Wilkies et al. 2013, p. 5). The main components of clinical scholarship described by the participants were: building and disseminating nursing knowledge, doing practice-based research, sharing knowledge, and linking academic research and practice, components seen to reflect the four dimensions of scholarship described by Boyer (1990) (Wilkies et al. 2013). Clinical scholarship is also a platform for thinking together, learn from each other's practice and in that way become capable practitioners. According to McDermott (1999) sharing knowledge involves guiding someone through our thinking or using our insights to help them see their own situations better.

Palmer (1986) traces the historical development of clinical scholarship over the span of a century of nursing incorporating the work of Nightingale. Nightingale's thinking about the nature and subject of observation became clear over time. In 1859 she advocated that nurses learn the physiognomy of disease (Nightingale 1859) and by 1882 she was publicising that, although observing the symptoms of illness was important, "it is, if possible, more important still, to observe the symptoms of nursing". And she declared the essential characteristics of clinical scholarship when she stated, "Observation tells us *how* the patient is; reflection tells us *what* is to be done; training tells us *how* it is to be done (Palmer 1986). Training and experience are, of course, necessary to teach us, too, *how* to observe; *how* to think; *what* to think. Observation tells us the fact; reflection, the meaning of the fact. Reflection needs training as much as observation" (Nightingale, 1882) (Palmer 1986, p. 319). Even before the concept of clinical scholarship had been articulated, Nightingale stipulated its components: observation, education, experience and intellectual activity (Palmer 1986, p. 319).

4.2.1   Definitions Surrounding the Milieu of Clinical Scholarship

Clinical scholarship is defined as that knowledge derived from the analysis and synthesis of observations of clients and patients, and is a complex activity that has as its purpose the discovery, organisation, analysis, synthesis, and transmission of knowledge resulting from client-oriented nursing practice (Palmer 1986). The observation, analysis, and synthesis of the phenomena with which professional nurses deal with in clinical nursing practice provide the matrix for clinical scholarship. This is not to imply that theoretical knowledge is excluded. Client-oriented nursing practice is an integration of theoretical and experiential knowledge (Palmer 1986, p. 318).

It is easier to discuss what clinical scholarship is not than what it is, it is not qualitative research, phenomenology or hermeneutics, not mere journalistic reporting or even the traditional case study (Diers 1995). Simply feeling, intuiting is not scholarship without informed, intelligent, imaginative, and clinically grounded analysis. In research, attention is paid to the numbers or concepts; in scholarship, care with the language is critical. In both cases, the activity is not complete until it is written down- the vital dissemination phase of generating knowledge (Diers 1995, p. 28). These principles are reinforced by Schlotfeldt (1992) who states that it is 'nursing's clinical scholarship that must be depended on to generate promising theories for testing that will advance nursing knowledge and ensure nursing's continued essential service to humankind' (p. 8).

Although clinical scholarship begins, as does clinical research, with observation, it builds differently (Diers 1995, p. 28). Excellent clinical research and scholarship share another potential similarity-they turn conventional ways of thinking upside down (Diers 2004, p. 86). Clinical research begins with a curiosity; clinical scholarship with the sense of wonder that we call "marvel". The satisfaction in clinical research comes with understanding what the data say, the satisfaction in scholarship comes in knowing (Diers 1995, p. 28). Besides, Vistinainer (1986) described two exemplar cases where the nurses observed, acted, and did the correct thing that in itself is not clinical scholarship. But the product of intellectual work that raises the clinical instance to the level of theory is a working draft on an idea about the world (Vistinainer 1986). As a working draft, theory is to be confronted and transformed by encounters with the real world of clinical work. That process is explicit in theory testing empirical research. It can be equally explicit in clinical scholarship. The clinical scholar must have a repertoire of possible explanations as well as the capacity to envision what the present instance *is an instance of* (Diers 2004, p. 85). Furthermore, clinical scholarship requires a maturity of practice that comes with experience and especially advanced specialist experience. Clinical scholarship is informed by reading, by thinking, by discussing with colleagues, by mentoring, by teaching so as to generate a mental map kit of potential explanations (Diers 2004, p. 87).

By virtue of their education and experience and clinical expertise, advanced practice nursing practitioners have a unique and significant part to play in advancing the development of nursing knowledge. Often believed to be the sole responsibility of academicians, clinical practice in essence is the field for knowledge development, for it is in the practice arena that nursing's phenomena of interest are encountered (Benner 1984; Benner et al. 1996). Knowledge development from a unique nursing perspective defines the boundaries of nursing and delineates the nature and application of nursing knowledge that explicates nurses' unique contribution to the health care team (Rolfe 2007). There is a need to create spaces for nurses to consider the nature of clinical scholarship, and how it could be enacted in the clinical milieu. In this way a further and vital contribution to the future of the discipline can be made, and a real commitment to excellence in clinical practice can be demonstrated (Wilkies et al. 2013).

The term clinical scholarship is one that has been used in nursing discourses over the recent past. Nurse academics have espoused that nursing must build a culture of clinical scholarship (Kitson 2006; Meleis 1992). Assuming an understanding of this form of scholarship without defining it, Mundinger et al. (2009) postulate that the 'cornerstone of clinical scholarship is the transfer of research to practice' (p. 73). Furthermore, in order to translate essential evidence-based knowledge into practice, the doctor of nursing graduate needs additional preparation in and knowledge of change processes, organisational systems, and evaluation methods. Practice change also entails using many skills that flow from practice relationships, communication, and collegial collaboration (Brown and Crabtree 2013, p. 336).

Academic scholarship has dominated the discourse in nursing. However, in order for nursing to develop and impact on health care, clinical scholarship needs to be explored and theorised. Nurse educators, hospital-based researchers and health organisations need to work together with academics to achieve this goal. Frameworks of scholarship conceptualised by nurse academics are reflected in the findings of a study with emphasis on reading and doing research and translating it into nursing practice which needs to be done in a non-threatening way (Wilkies et al. 2013). As revealed in that study, clinical scholarship develops from learning from other's research, reading research and putting research findings into practice, conducting systematic reviews, developing the scholar nurse's own research, developing collaborative research and doing research from the scholar's own practice base (Wilkies et al. 2013).

In order to develop and nurture clinical scholarship, an enabling research culture within the health care arena and the academy must be developed to capture and sustain the creativity of the advanced practice nursing practitioner/aspirant. This culture needs to be categorised by research productivity, positive interprofessional collegial relationships, inclusivity and effective research processes and training. The health care arena must provide a safe environment for clinicians to discuss and theorise about clinical scholarship (Dopson 2007). As well, health care organisations and nurse leaders in these organisations must encourage and build structures such as practice development projects with a focus on improving patient care (Kitson 2006; McCormack and McCance 2006), by encouraging and assisting clinical nurses to pursue research and its translation back to practice (Wilkies et al. 2013).

Advanced practice nursing practitioners can earn the rites-to-passage towards becoming a scholar-practitioner (see Fig. 4.1). The spectrum [landscape] of clinical scholarship model incorporates five dimensions of scholarship with specific indicators identified within each. Some of the indicators within the five dimensions may overlap. The definitions provided by Boyer have been incorporated to inform the indicators within each of the scholarship dimensions; Scholarship of Engagement, Scholarship of Integration, Scholarship of Application, Scholarship of Discovery and Scholarship of Teaching. The three characteristics associated reciprocally with

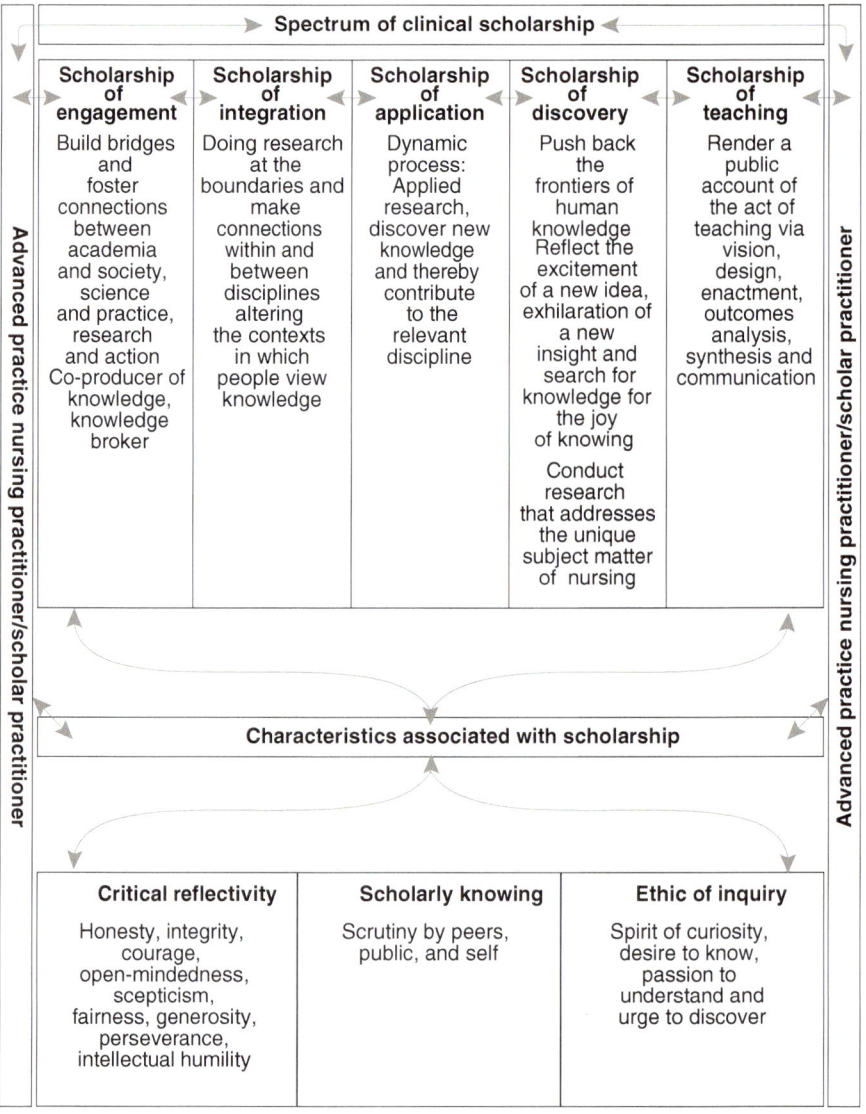

Fig. 4.1 Spectrum of clinical scholarship model

scholarship weave through each of the dimensions and are exclusive to each of the dimensions, but yet collectively inform all five dimensions while connecting with and relating to the scholarly activity of the advanced practice nursing practitioner/ scholar practitioner (see Fig. 4.1). Moreover, the three characteristics; critical reflectivity, scholarly knowing, and ethic of inquiry and their identifiers act as a platform to construct and transform the scholarly activity of the advanced practice nursing practitioner within the context of engagement, integration, application, discovery and teaching into clinical scholarship.

Building a community of scholar-practitioners requires the development of a research culture within organisations that employ nurses and an environment that builds a sense of community. A community of scholar-practitioners in nursing inseparably linked with the community of patients/service users and families that we serve, is a vision for the future of the nursing profession. Nurses will then be speaking for nursing, partnered with patients and focused on health (Ferguson-Pare 2005). There are some similarities with the philosophy of developing a research culture with the portrayal of establishing a person-centered culture. According to McCormack et al. (2015) establishing a person-centered culture requires a sustained commitment to practice developments, service improvements and ways of working that embrace continuous feedback, reflection and engagement methods that enable all voices to be heard (p. 3). Patient-centred approaches to care are altering the future landscape of healthcare and the role of the advanced practice nursing practitioner/aspirant is central to sustaining this partnership in practice aligned with a culture that nurtures the structures, processes and outcomes warranted in such a clinical milieu.

4.2.2 Patient Centered Care

The current focus on patient-centered care (PCC) approaches endeavours to redress imbalances in health care and represents a shift from the previous approach that was medically dominated and disease oriented. The PCC approach seeks to establish collaborative partnerships and adopts a holistic approach that strives to meet and acknowledge patients' values, preferences, and expressed needs while enhancing their engagement and involvement in decisions. This approach is inherent in many of nursing care theories such as Leininger's (1988) theory of culture care, Boykin and Schoenhofer's (1993) theory of nursing as caring, Roach's (1987) conceptualisation of caring relationships (Delaney 2018, p. 121) and Meehan's careful nursing model (Meehan 2003).

Nurses have the capacity to support and assist in the meaningful improvement and operationalisation of PCC (McCormack and McCance 2017; McCance 2003). Transformational leadership, innovative practices (e.g., respecting patient choices) and collaborative approaches have been adopted to meet the needs of patients and improve the provision of health care and consumer satisfaction with the care provided (Edwards et al. 2004). These approaches identify the critical humanistic role of nurses in collaborating with patients and promoting and advocating for their patients' choices and represent a need to move beyond technical competencies in the provision of health care (Delaney 2018, pp. 121–122). Increasing specialisation and divergent professional paths mean that a single healthcare professional, no matter how talented or skilled, cannot subsist alone, building teams with diverse competencies is essential to fulfil patients' needs (Sakallaris et al. 2016, p. 57).

For those who agree that patient-centeredness should be a part of nursing identity in practice, Bell et al. (2015) reported that there is a need for development of health services research into both the nature of caring construct in nursing identity and its expression in practice. Computational text analytics software was used to analyse all health services abstracts in the database PubMed since 1986. Abstracts were treated as indicative of the content of health services research. A total of 234,926 abstracts were obtained. Leximancer software was used in 1) mapping of 4,144,458 instances of 107 concepts; 2) analysis of 106 paired concept co-occurrences for the nursing concept; and 3) sentiment analysis of the nursing concept versus patient, family and community concepts, and clinical concepts (Bell et al. 2015, p. 1). The findings reveal that nursing is constructed within quality assurance or service implementation or workforce development concepts. It is relatively disconnected from patient, family and community concepts and clinical concepts (Bell et al. 2015, p. 1). This study raises some important questions for the discipline of health services research, as well as nursing advocacy, research and education. It suggests that a key evidence-base for health services—PubMed—tends not to position nurses as patient-centered caregivers. In so doing, Bell et al.'s study contributes to broad popular and scholarly debates about whether the nursing profession needs to actively re-appropriate constructs of patient care as more central to nursing identity. More fundamentally, the study raises questions about whether health services research cultures even value the politically popular idea of nurses as patient-centered caregivers, as this growing scholarly discipline enters the twenty-first century, and whether they should be valued in this context (Bell et al. 2015, p. 13).

Bell et al. (2015) further expands on the findings; the disconnect of nursing from technical clinical concepts as well as more technical epidemiological concepts potentially jeopardises nursing identity in two other critical ways. That is, the disconnect of nursing from clinical concepts could be seen as suggesting a repositioning of nurses as subordinate to clinical experts (Bell et al. 2015, p. 13). In addition, the most ambiguous findings lie in the sentiment analysis and raises important questions. Is the relative marginalisation of nursing in health services research, away from the central patient concept, as well as dominant clinical concepts, somehow caused by or leading to the use of the nursing concept in less positive ways? That is, put colloquially, is taking the care out of nursing linked to not caring about nursing? (Bell et al. 2015, p. 13). Earlier, Lutz and Bowers (2000) urged nurses to throw off medical authority and embrace the distinct, patient-centred heritage of nursing. They present PCC as a source of not only in-group superiority but potential in-group advantage. 'With its long-standing commitment to being patient focused, nursing is in a prime position to lead the research effort [on] patient-centred models of care' (p. 179). Surprisingly, their concept of PCC hinges on a 'philosophical shift … from providing care for patients to providing services to consumers' (Lutz and Bowers, p. 173). The interaction between nurse and patient is central to the effective study and application of PCC. According to Hobbs (2009) appropriate use of PCC can improve study outcomes and measurements by clarifying the variables involved, and PCC holds great promise to frame patient outcome and satisfaction research by analyzing how and with what effect nurses alleviate patient vulnerability. Moreover, consideration of information practices as a critical supporting structure of nurse-patient interaction can be explored (Hobbs 2009).

The increasing specialisation of medicine and nursing, in the context of a continuous striving for greater efficiency, has reduced contact time between individual patients and individual members of staff (Goodrich and Cornwell 2008, p. 2). "Quality" in health care and medical care has two distinct connotations. One has to do with professional competence, the technical quality of diagnostic and therapeutic procedures and equipment, the appropriateness of treatment, and the efficiency of the systems that deliver this care. The quality of the patient's experience, however, is something else again, and this can be assessed only by patients themselves (Gerteis et al. 1993, p. 2). Consequently, the Picker/Commonwealth Program for Patient-Centered Care set out in 1987 to explore patients' needs and concerns, as patients themselves define them (Gerteis et al. 1993). They conducted focus groups with patients and members of their families, reviewed the literature and consulted other health professionals and identified seven broad "dimensions" of care that most affect patients' experiences:

1. Respect for patients' values, preferences and expressed needs;
2. Coordination of care and integration of services within an institutional setting;
3. Communication between patient and providers; dissemination of accurate, timely and appropriate information; and education about the long-term implications of disease and illness;
4. Physical care, comfort and the alleviation of pain;
5. Emotional support and alleviation of fears and anxiety;
6. Involvement of family and friends; and
7. Transition and continuity from one locus of care to another (Gerteis et al. 1993, p. 2).

Then, a survey instrument was designed to elicit reports from patients about concrete aspects of their experience within the seven broad dimensions of care, in lieu of the satisfaction ratings generally used on patient surveys (Gerteis et al. 1993, p. 3). In 1989, more than 6000 recently hospitalised patients were interviewed, randomly selected from 62 hospitals nationwide, along with 2999 of the friends or family members who served as their "care partners". More than 20 hospitals were also visited, including those identified as "exemplary" by professionals in the field and hospitals that scored high or low on the national survey (Gerteis et al. 1993, p. 3).

The survey (Gerteis et al. 1993) had four main purposes; 1) to determine the magnitude of the problem; 2) to identify the dimensions of care; 3) to identify groups of patients "at risk" and 4) to determine, in broad terms, the institutional characteristics that affect patients' experiences. Of the patients interviewed, 80% rated their care "excellent" or "very good". Yet, behind these aggregate ratings, actual experiences varied markedly, according to the experts elicited in the survey, reflecting wide differences among demographic groups, institutions and particular dimensions of care (Gerteis et al. 1993, p. 3). One of the most compelling themes to emerge from the patient focus groups conducted early in the Picker/Commonwealth project is that what patients seem to care most about are not the things health professionals often think they care about. What loomed large in patients' mind were the sense of vulnerability and helplessness that illness and hospitalisation created and the dependency on others, even, at times, for help with the most routine activities of daily living. Until those basic needs were met, patients could focus on little else (Gerteis et al. 1993, p. 5).

4.2.3 Definitions and Dimensions of Patient-Centered Care

There is considerable ambiguity concerning the exact meaning of the term and the optimum method of measuring the process and outcomes of patient-centered care.

The most comprehensive description is provided by Stewart et al. (1995) whose model of patient-centered care identified six interconnecting components:

1. Exploring both the disease and the illness experience;
2. Understanding the whole person;
3. Finding common ground regarding management;
4. Incorporating prevention and health promotion;
5. Enhancing the doctor-patient relationship;
6. Being realistic about personal limitations and issues such as the availability of time and resources.

To date, the term 'patient-centeredness' has been used to denote to so many diverse concepts that its scientific value may have been compromised. The proposed "five-dimension framework; 'biopsychosocial perspective'; 'person-as-person'; 'sharing power and responsibility'; 'therapeutic alliance'; and 'doctor-as-person', each representing a particular aspect of the relationship between doctor and patient provides conceptual clarity concerning the exact issues addressed by particular interventions or research tools should facilitate communication between different research groups, and between researchers and clinicians" (Mead and Bower 2000, p. 1103).

The Institute of Medicine (IOM) (2001) defined patient-centered care as care that is respectful of and responsive to individual patient preferences, needs, and values. Following a series of focus groups with patients, iterative feedback from research colleagues and consultation with rational advisors, Greene et al. (2012) modified the IOM definition slightly to describe patient-centered care as care that "honours and responds to individual patient preferences, needs, values, and goals". It is through this lens that they describe why and how patient-centered care should be an imperative for all health care systems, whether that "system" is a solo practitioner, a large multispeciality group practice, or a federally qualified health center providing care to underserved populations (Greene et al. 2012, p. 49). The World Health Organisation also promoted a person-centered approach, with a global goal of humanising healthcare by ensuring that it is rooted in universal principles of human rights and dignity, non-discrimination, participation and empowerment, access and equity, and a partnership of equals:

> *The overall vision for people-centered health care services "… an approach to care that consciously adopts the perspectives of individuals, families and communities and sees them as participants as well as beneficiaries of trusted health systems that respond to their needs and preferences in humane and holistic ways…* (World Health Organisation 2015, p. 10).

Based on a scoping review (n = 101 articles) Constand et al. (2014) reported a lack of consistency between the meaning of health promotion within patient-centered care and other aspects of healthcare. They suggest a specific definition would improve this component of patient centered care. For example, health promotion has been defined by the World Health Organisation as the process of enabling people to increase control over their health and its determinants, and thereby improve their health (WHO, 1986). However, within the patient-centered care literature it has been defined as developing healthcare plans based on reflection on patient histories for the purposes of health enhancement, risk reduction, and early detection of illness (Little et al. 2001). The patient-centered care definition implicitly refers to the clinical interaction and goals; whereas, the World Health Organisation places greater emphasis on determinants of health. Differences in conceptual framing of health promotion make it difficult to isolate studies that investigate the effect of this component of patient-centered care on outcomes (Constand et al. 2014).

A systematic review was conducted of patient-centered care (PCC) literature to examine the evidence for PCC and outcomes. Three databases (Medline, CINAHL, PsycINFO) were searched for all years through September 2012 and 40 articles out of a total of 1218 articles were retained for the analysis (Rathert et al. 2012). A wide range of methodologies was represented, from quasi-experimental, randomised designs, to longitudinal, multimethod studies, cross-sectional surveys and qualitative interview designs. Studies took place in a variety of countries, indicating that PCC is a topic of international interest (Rathert et al. 2012).

Overall the literature on PCC processes and outcomes portrayed generally positive empirical relationships between PCC and intermediate as well as some distal outcomes (Rathert et al. 2012). Although the randomised studies found mixed results for long-term clinical outcomes, some of these studies did find positive relationships. Most of the non-randomised longitudinal studies did find relationships between PCC and clinical outcomes. These studies were more likely to account for variability of PCC from providers, and as well, capture a broader spectrum of the patient experience (Rathert et al. 2012, p. 373). Almost all studies, regardless of methodology, found positive relationships between PCC processes and patient satisfaction and well-being. This is important for two reasons. First, patient satisfaction with the care experience has become an important outcome in its own right. Second, some research suggests that patient well-being and satisfaction may be related to mediating variables, such as adherence and self-management behaviours (Rathert et al. 2012, pp. 373–374).

According to Quatrara and Dale Shaw (2017) most institutions routinely measure patient satisfaction in a global manner. Like other aggregate data, it is hard to specifically attribute the outcomes to advanced practice registered nurses (APRN) practice. For example, in many cases, the satisfaction instrument will not distinguish the APRN from the bedside nurse or the physician. Further complicating the matter, many institutions collect data related only to the service line (i.e., medicine or surgery). Thus for satisfaction to be linked to APRN practice, a separate survey may be necessary (Quatrara and Dale Shaw 2017). These findings should resonate with advanced practice nursing practitioners/aspirants pertinent to capturing appropriate data on the patient experience in order to provide specific evidence of their unique contribution to and impact on patient care outcomes.

There was a notable lack of research focused specifically on the dimensions of co-ordination of care, emotional support, physical comfort, continuity and transition, while none of the PCC studies in the review examined involvement of the family (Rathert et al. 2012). This is particularly notable given that families provide extensive informal care and play an important role in the patient's psychosocial context, particularly in chronic disease and older-person care. Co-ordination of care was only directly examined in two studies, and physical comfort was only examined in one study. Although these dimensions were indicated as components of PCC by the IOM (2001) and the Picker Institute, they have perhaps in the literature been examined as concepts or variables in their own right as opposed to components of PCC (Rathert et al. 2012, p. 374).

Present models and definitions of patient-centeredness revealed a lack of conceptual clarity. Based on a prior systematic review, Zill et al. (2015) developed an integrative model with 15 dimensions of patient-centeredness. The aims of this study was to 1) validate, and 2) prioritise these dimensions (p. 1). A two-round web-based Delphi study was conducted. 297 international experts were invited to participate. In round one they were asked to 1) give an individual rating on a nine-point-scale on relevance and clarity of the dimensions, 2) add missing dimensions, and 3) prioritise the dimensions in Delphi round 2, experts received feedback about the results of round 1 and were asked to reflect and re-rate their own results. The cut-off for the validation of a dimension was a median < 7 on one of the criteria.

One hundred and five experts (clinicians, patient representatives, researchers and quality managers) participated in Delphi round one and 71 in Delphi round 2. Based on the results of the Delphi survey, Zill et al. (2015) presented a revision of the original model including the relevance and clarity rating of the experts. In this model they aligned their 15 dimensions of patient-centered care to three categories namely a) *principles*, b) *enablers* and c) *activities*. This proposed differentiation showed the interrelation of the dimensions. Zill et al. (2015) found the dimensions *patient as a unique person*, *biopsychosocial perspective*, *essential characteristics of the clinician* and *clinician-patient relationship* as the underlying *principles* of a patient-centered (p. 10) care model (Zill et al. 2015, p. 11).

One of the *enablers*, namely *physician-patient communication* was rated as one of the five most important dimensions. From the four dimensions that were labelled as *principles* of patient-centeredness, *patient as a unique person* was rated as the most important dimension and the dimension *biopsychosocial perspective* was judged to be insufficiently clear. Those dimensions described as patient-centered *activities* all reached sufficiently high ratings and three were considered in the top five rating of importance (Zill et al. 2015, p. 11). Overall, the model provides a useful framework that can be used in the development of measures, interventions, and medical education curricula, as well as the adoption of a new perspective in health policy (Zill et al. 2015, pp. 1–2).

Despite widespread belief in the importance of patient-centred care, it remains difficult to create a system in which all groups work together for the good of the patient/client. Part of the problem may be that the issue of patient-centred care itself can be used to prosecute intergroup conflict (Kreindler 2013). A qualitative study of texts examined the presence and nature of intergroup language within the discourse on patient-centred care. A systematic SCOPUS and Google search identified 85 peer-reviewed and grey literature reports that engaged with the concept of patient-centred care. Discourse analysis, informed by the social identity approach, examined how writers defined and portrayed various groups (Kreindler 2013). In addition, a systematic search was conducted for English-language reports that engaged with the concept of PCC and/or the question of how to achieve it. The intent was not to assemble a complete body of relevant literature, but to derive a sample of reports reflecting the main perspectives from which PCC has been addressed (Kreindler 2013, p. 1141).

The results reported that managers, physicians and nurses all used the discourse of patient-centred care to imply that their own group was patient centred while other group(s) were not. Patient organisations tended to downplay or even deny the role of managers and providers in promoting patient centeredness, and some used the concept to advocate for controversial health policies. Intergroup themes were even more obvious in the rhetoric of political groups across the ideological spectrum. In contrast to accounts that juxtaposed in-groups and out-groups, those from reportedly patient-centred organisations defined a 'mosaic' in-group that encompassed managers, providers and patients (Kreindler 2013). The seemingly benign concert of patient-centred care can easily become a weapon on an intergroup battlefield. Of note, understanding this dimension may help organisations resolve the intergroup tensions that prevent collective achievement of a patient-centred system (Kreindler 2013, p. 1139).

Health care professionals present the aspiration towards patient centeredness as grounded in professional identity, envisioning patient- or person-centred care in terms of humanistic values and partnership, not consumerism and buyer-seller relationships. Indeed, they can lead the charge for patient centeredness, understood as a fuller expression of their professional identity (Irvine 2004). The problem however, arises when professional groups use this genuine and legitimate aspect of identity content to buttress the claim that they are already patient centred—and others are not (Kreindler 2013, p. 1143).

Healing relationships have an underlying structure and lead to important patient-centered outcomes (Scott et al. 2008). Clinicians often have an intuitive understanding of how their relationships with patients foster healing. Yet little is empirically known about the experience of healing and how it occurs between clinicians and patients. Scott et al. (2008) attempted to create a model that identified how healing relationships are developed and maintained. Primary care clinicians (n = 6) were purposefully selected as exemplar healers. Patients (n = 23) were selected by these clinicians as having experienced healing relationships. In-depth interviews, designed to elicit stories of healing relationships, were conducted with patients and clinicians separately (Scott et al. 2008).

Three key processes emerged as fostering healing relationships: (1) valuing/creating a non-judgemental emotional bond; (2) appreciating power/consciously managing clinician power in ways that would most benefit the patient; and (3) abiding/displaying a commitment to caring for patients over time. Three relational outcomes resulted from these processes: trust, hope and a sense of being known. Clinician competencies that facilitate these processes are self-confidence, emotional self-management, mindfulness, and knowledge (Scott et al. 2008). Exemplar clinicians (n = 6) reported that most often they work to increase patients' power. One way they do this is by engaging patients as partners. Another way of managing power is to educate patients by translating medical jargon into language patients understand and by providing patients with the knowledge needed to manage their own illnesses.

Sometimes, however, clinicians carefully pushed resistant patients to take actions that were important to their health (Scott et al. 2008, p. 318). Exemplar clinicians described an intuitive understanding about when and how to push patients based on assessments of patients' needs and strength of relationships. One physician described it this way "… sometimes you're the coach and sometimes you're the boss and sometimes you're the sibling and sometimes you're the doctor" (Scott et al. 2008, p. 318). Clinician-patient healing relationships have discernible structure and lead to patient-centered outcomes. This conceptual model of clinician-patient healing relationships may be generalizable to other kinds of healing relationships (Scott et al. 2008, p. 320). In nursing, a focus on the whole person and the relationship between nurse and patient are both central and primary to both the processes and outcomes of practice (Quinn et al. 2003, p. A65).

Person-centered care requires clinicians skilled in relationship building, empathy, compassion and clinicians who can work well in interdisciplinary teams (Sakallaris et al. 2016, p. 56). Person-centered care requires professional artistry and is developed through learner-centered education that is transformative and incorporates a framework of reflective practice (Sakallaris et al. 2016, p. 57). Person-centered care cannot be implemented with a one-off 'quick fix' (Manley and McCormack 2008) but requires a change in the values of both the acute healthcare system and individual practitioners (Kontos and Naglie 2007). Of note, Richards et al. (2015, p. 3) suggest that it is 'time to get real about delivering person-centered care' and maintain that this requires a sea change in the mind-set of health professionals and patients/clients alike. McCormack et al. (2013) argue that a significant part of this sea change is the need to shift the discourse away from person-centered 'care' per se and to promote a unified discourse of person-centered 'cultures'. Person-centeredness can only happen if there is a person-centered culture in place in care settings that enables staff to experience person-centeredness and work in a person-centered way. With a focus on person-centered culture, the authors adopt the following definition of person-centeredness:

> … An approach to practice established through the formation and fostering of healthful relationships between all care providers, service users and others significant to them in their lives. It is underpinned by values of respect for persons, individual right to self-determination, mutual respect and understanding. It is enabled by cultures of empowerment that foster continuous approaches to practice development (McCormack et al. 2013, p. 193).

Sakallaris et al. (2016) proposed three requirements that are necessary when person-centered is hardwired into practice: (1) policy changes that incentivise healthcare systems, clinicians and patients for providing and utilising primary care, preventative, and self-care health promotion activities; (2) systematic inclusion of patients and family perspectives in healthcare system decisions, best practice evidence generation and clinical education; and (3) learner-centric clinical education that integrates relationship skill building with the scientific curricula (Sakallaris et al. 2016, p. 59). Moreover, communication is part of the person centered practice agenda.

Patient-centered communication has been defined mainly from the viewpoint of *physicians'* behaviours to achieve patient-centered care (McCormack et al. 2011; Epstein et al. 2005; Stewart et al. 2003; Stewart 2000). It is typically the physicians who are asked to modify their orientation to achieve patient-centered care, with the patient behaviours being less often discussed. This may be due to the implicit assumption that patients are vulnerable in the relationship with the physician and thus need to be protected (Ishikawa et al. 2013, p. 151).

One such vulnerable population are people with dementia. There are seven core ideas which are consistently identified as essential to the practice of person-centered care for people with dementia: (1) addressing the person's social environment to support their personhood; (2) acknowledging the uniqueness of the person; (3) respecting autonomy, dignity and rights of the person; (4) focusing on the person's strengths and positive aspects rather than deficits and weaknesses; (5) valuing the person's perspective and subjective experiences; (6) valuing and supporting care staff and other stakeholders to co-construct a caring relationship; (7) and enabling the person to enact and build on continuing opportunities for agency (Poland and Birt 2016; Edvardsson et al. 2010; Hughes et al. 2008; Brooker 2004; Kitwood 1997). Using Kitwood's five dimensions of personhood; identity, inclusion, attachment, comfort and occupation as an *priori* framework, Clissett et al. (2013) explored the way in which current approaches to care in acute settings had the potential to enhance personhood in older adults with dementia. Participants were people aged over 70 on acute wards in two major hospitals in the UK, identified through a screening process as having possible mental health problems. 34 patients and their relatives were recruited: this analysis focused on the 29 patients with cognitive impairment. Data collection involved 72 hours of ward-based non-participant observations of care complemented by 30 formal interviews after discharge concerning the experiences of care of the 29 patients with cognitive impairment (Clissett et al. 2013).

The findings revealed a number of strategies deployed by healthcare workers appeared to have the net result of giving a sense of inclusion to the person-with-dementia, taking opportunities for engagement with the person-with-dementia; demonstrating that the welfare of the person was important; and ensuring that they were involved in making key decisions about their future. A key element in making people-with-dementia feel included was involvement in key decisions illustrated by the patient and family member while facing a major decision about future care:

> We went into a small room. There was my brother, myself – my mother was with us because they said she was the person that was concerned she had to be there ... he said even though she may not understand what we're talking about, all of it, she has the right to be there because it concerns her. And we talked about it, there was a nurse, the doctor, my brother, myself and my mother, and that was the first time that had happened (Clissett et al. 2013, p. 1499).

Therefore person-centered care needs to re-focus dementia care from person-hood providing the moral imperative to care, to supporting that person to remain a citizen with social standing within their community with a stronger voice in their own care (Poland and Birt 2016).

Patient-centered care is about forensically unravelling the narrative in each clinical encounter, an activity that is core to the advanced practice nursing practitioners' inventory (O'Connor et al. 2018). Although previous studies have directed less attention to patient competencies in communicating with the health-care provider (Clayman et al. 2010), patient centered communication cannot be achieved if patients are unwilling or unable to fulfil the roles identified. Growing attention to patient health literacy—"the capacity to obtain, process and understand basic health information and services needed to make appropriate health decisions" (Selden et al. 2000, p. vi)—in health communication research may correspond to this conceptualisation of patient-centered communication (McManus et al. 2017). Furthermore, although patient-centered communication has been defined mainly from the viewpoint of *physicians'* behaviours, aimed at achieving patient-centered care, patient competence is also required for patient-centered communication, and this should be explored in current medical practice (Ishikawa et al. 2013, p. 152). Furthermore, in the empowerment discourse 'information for choice'—rather than 'information for compliance'—is considered an important patient right (Pulvirenti et al. 2014; Henwood et al. 2003). It is argued that, if patients lack "health literacy skills", then this ability to "critically analyse information" needs to be built by healthcare professionals and/or the broader healthcare system (Pulvirenti et al. 2014).

The essence of patient-centered care necessitates that the advanced practice nursing practitioner/aspirant views the health care experience through the patient's eyes. Equally, shared decision-making is part of this process, that depends on building a good relationship in the clinical encounter so that information is shared and patients are supported to deliberate and express their preferences and views during the decision making process. According to Barry and Edgman-Levitan (2012) we will have succeeded in building a truly patient-centered health care system when an informed woman can decide whether to have a screening mammogram and an informed man can consider whether to have a screening prostate-specific-antigen test without their clinicians labelling the decision "wrong" on the basis of different values and preferences (p. 781). To accomplish these tasks, Elwyn et al. (2010, 2012) proposed a model of how to do shared decision making that is based on *choice, option* and *decision talk*. The model has three steps: a) introducing choice, b) describing options, often by integrating the use of patient decision support tools, and c) helping patients explore preferences and make decisions. This model rests on supporting a process of deliberation, and on understanding that decisions should be influenced by exploring and respecting "what matters most" to patients as individuals, and that this exploration in turn depends on them developing informed preferences and the use of decision support tools provide crucial inputs into this process (Elwyn et al. 2012, p. 1363). That said, Jayadevappa and Chhatre (2011) argue that patient-centered care is about tailored care, which means that physicians and nurses accept that some patients prefer to actively participate in decision-making, while others opt for a more passive role and wish to defer decisions to their physicians (O'Connor 2016). Therefore, cultural competence needs to be factored into patient-centered care so that healthcare professionals understand and are responsive to patient beliefs, preferences and needs, and consequently build rapport and trust (Jayadevappa and Chhatre 2011).

Healthcare acknowledges the importance of patient-centered approaches, including paying attention to patient views' on care (Curry et al. 2005; Stewart 2001; Cromarty 1996; Cameron-Traub 1995). Clinical empathy includes three components: (1) understanding a patient's situation and how the patients feels about it; (2) communicating this understanding and checking with the patient to assess accuracy of interpretation; and (3) using this understanding to help the patient address the issue at hand (Mercer and Reynolds 2002). The empathetic activities of the advanced practice nursing practitioner pertain to the seven dimensions that affect the patient experience in the clinical setting outlined by Gerteis et al. (1993). That said, metrics and key performance indicators associated with those broad patient-centered dimensions need to be captured through research by the advanced practice nursing practitioners so that their contributions are visible, and accessible for scrutiny by self, peers, the public and the patient/service-user. In addition, critical reflection, creativity and active learning, using the conceptual ideas underpinning person-centered care and practice development underpins the design and implementation of the advanced practice professional capabilities portfolio (see Chap. 6) that is much needed to create and sustain such cultures of scholarly practice (LeGrow and Espin 2017).

Consequently, community engagement is an opportunity for advanced practice nursing practitioners/aspirants to learn about community members' individual experiences, as personal stories provide useful information for health impact assessment reports, and also help personalise population health issues. By learning about others' experiences, we see the world through another's perspective, which is key for developing empathy (Chinchilla and Arcaya 2017) and an important concept in patient-centered care. Communities of Practice align with the Scholarship of Engagement advocated by Boyer (1996) and can also align with making healthcare more patient-centered in the context of the advanced practice nursing practitioner's policy context agenda.

4.2.4   Communities of Practice Support A Culture of Clinical Scholarship

Advanced practice nursing practitioners are trained and educated through hands-on activities that focus on understanding the complexities of practice. Understanding these complexities that tackle the intricacies of community development and policy context is important. In addition, the public health's objective of addressing health inequalities gives advanced practice nursing practitioners a clear goal. Both health care planners and public health experts recognise the importance of community engagement, and that addressing health disparities requires practitioners assurance that previously marginalised communities have a seat at the decision-making table. Hence, advanced practice nursing practitioners need to interact with community members, including patients/service-users and families in order to engage these key stakeholders in project decisions, and attend community meetings and interact with key stakeholders through site visits.

According to Wenger (1998) Communities of Practice (CoPs) members' negotiation of meanings in practice leads to the development of three structural elements of CoPs: (i) mutual engagement (how and what people do together as part of practice), (ii) joint enterprise (a set of problems and topics that they care about), and (iii) shared repertoire (the concepts and artefacts that they create). More recent work by Pyrko et al. (2017) reported that the process of 'thinking together' is conceptualised as a key part of meaningful Communities of Practice where academics and practitioners mutually guide each other through their understandings of the same problems in their area of mutual interest, and in this way directly share tacit knowledge. The collaborative learning process of 'thinking together', they argue is what essentially brings Communities of Practice to life and not the other way around (Pyrko et al. 2017, p. 389).

The advanced practice nursing practitioner has much to gain engaging within Communities of Practice towards meeting the criteria of clinical scholarship. In this scenario participants from different settings are no longer merely insiders and outsiders but stakeholders working toward shared purposes who can accomplish more together than they might accomplish separately. In this way the spectrum of clinical scholarship (see Fig. 4.1) and its critical elements associated with the characteristics of scholarship of engagement, integration, application, discovery and teaching could be the visionary step in populating elements of the declared legacy map portfolio (see Chap. 6).

Communities of Practice are collectively engaged in the creation of new ideas and innovations and connect scholars across institutions, leveraging collective analysis of a problem to create an innovative solution. Hence, a Community of Practice is defined as a collaborative, informal network that supports professional practitioners in their efforts to develop shared understandings and engage in work-relevant knowledge building (Confessore 1997). Participation involves more than networking or exchanging data. Junior members can be fostered via legitimate peripheral participation, progressively developing abilities that allow greater contribution over time (Sherbino et al. 2010). This is where those rich social networks discussed by Brown and Duguid come into play. The aforementioned authors argued, it is not the availability of information itself that is key, but active participation in Communities of Practice. "Become a member of a community, engage in its practices, you can acquire and make use of its knowledge and information" (Brown and Duguid 2000, p. 126). From this perspective, the key to demand for pedagogical knowledge-including what is produced by practitioners through the scholarship of teaching and learning-is the expansion of Communities of Practice around teaching and learning itself (Huber 2009, p. 4).

Boyer's definition of the scholarship of engagement makes reference to outreach as a communal act. But its uniqueness is that as an activity, outreach is also a communal process (Bruns et al. 2003, p. 7). For outreach to have the largest impact, the partnership between the university and community must be reciprocal. Outreach is not an end product. It is a part of a circular process by which what is learned is then incorporated into the other aspects of our work, work that subsequently impacts our engagement with the community (Bruns et al. 2003, p. 9). For communities, which have an abundance of opportunities that are challenging and thought-provoking, the "real value" of engagement appears in discovery through applied research and action research. Hence action research, when conducted in partnership with the community by advanced practice nursing practitioners adds to the knowledge base of the discipline, while at the same time providing the community with valuable research-based information that can help formulate policy decisions that have long-term impact on citizens.

Central to understanding outreach as scholarly expression is respecting it as a complex phenomenon. First, outreach is expressed in many ways, not a one-size-fits all. Second, the very word *outreach* conveys a distinct epistemological, ontological, and axiological reference point (Fear et al. 2001). "Reaching out is academy-centered (knowledge from) and unidirectional (to those who benefit). Other terms used in the field, such as service and *engagement*, are challenging for a different reason: the words have diffuse meaning and are open to multiple interpretations. Who is serving and engaging whom? Why? How? Under what circumstances? Towards what ends?" (Fear et al. 2001, p. 22).

Thinking of outreach as a complex phenomenon has theoretical and practical value; firstly, it keeps academics from embracing the notion that there is a definitive outreach expression or a best form for undertaking it, because with an incredible array of problems, situations, settings, and challenges facing us in the outreach domain, it is impractical and even dangerous to endorse a "one size fits all" way of thinking (Fear et al. 2001, p. 23). Academics need to adjust their research and practice to the realities of the setting as they experience it which necessitates approaching outreach as a form of inquiry. Secondly, Smith (1997) proposed viewing outreach as complex compels academics to keep on the look-out for new expressions and forms, such as participatory action research (PAR). According to Bryant-Lukosious et al. (2017) the principles of participatory action research (PAR) are relevant to the advanced practice nursing (APN) role development. APN practitioners work collaboratively within interprofessional teams and in established relationships with other stakeholders in the health system. Stakeholder roles and relationships are influenced by their values, beliefs, experiences, and expectations. These relationships create the conditions that impact the effective delivery of health services and yet can also facilitate or obstruct the implementation of APN roles (Bryant-Lukosious et al. 2017).

The engagement boundary is a place where academics and advanced practice nursing practitioners/aspirants advance in their understanding of outreach as a dynamic and evolving phenomenon. It is in this regard that *reflexivity* matters, which means turning the investigative lens on self in critically recursive ways as though the self is "the other" and that means seeking to better appreciate and understand our dynamic and evolving scholarly selves (Fear et al. 2001, p. 29). Engaging in reflective practice is one of the norms of engagement. It is among many approaches and practices with "alternative paradigm inquiry", including qualitative and participatory approaches and scholars need to recognise, understand, and respect multiple ways of knowing, interpreting, and practicing (Fear and Sandmann 2001–2002). Moreover, service-learning is one of the many contemporary examples of scholarly "boundary   crossings"   ways   that   faculty   connect—in   scholarly   ways—the traditionally discrete activities of teaching, research and service, and viewed in this way, engagement becomes a connective expression (Fear and Sandmann 2001–2002). That happens when the preposition "of" (the scholarship of engagement) is replaced with the preposition "in" and when that occurs, engagement becomes a cross-cutting phenomenon—engagement in teaching, in research, and in service—guided by an engagement ethos (Fear and Sandmann 2001–2002).

Communities of Practice aligned with the scholarship of engagement advocated by Boyer could raise the profile of person-centered care and embrace the deeper meaning of person-centeredness rather than only the adoption of the term person-centered care. In developing person-centeredness and person-centered care, scholarship comprising research, teaching and service to the community characterised by integrity in the practices of systematic enquiry and discovery; a willingness to create interprofessional connections across scholarly domains, and evaluate complex interventions, would provide a platform enabling advanced practice nursing practitioners produce credible scholarship for the discipline and the people they serve in a variety of complex clinical milieus.

4.3   Conclusion

Clinical scholarship exists along a continuum of evidence-based practice, quality improvement and research. Advanced practice nursing practitioners' active involvement in clinical scholarship is necessary to advance the nursing profession and improve patient outcomes. Clinical scholarship was defined as that knowledge derived from the analysis and synthesis of observations of patients, a complex activity that has as its purpose the discovery, integration, application, engagement and knowledge translation in clinical practice. Simply feeling, intuiting is not scholarship without informed, intelligent, and clinically grounded analysis. In order to develop and nurture clinical scholarship, an enabling research culture within the healthcare arena and the academy must be developed to capture and sustain the creativity of the advanced practice nursing practitioner/aspirant. This culture needs to be categorised by research productivity, positive interprofessional collegial relationships, inclusivity and effective research processes and training.

Advanced practice nursing practitioners can earn the rites-to-passage towards being a scholar-practitioner. The spectrum [landscape] of clinical scholarship model was illustrated (see Fig. 4.1) that incorporates five dimensions of scholarship with specific indicators identified within each. The qualities associated with a scholar practitioner that merit special consideration in the context of scholarship: integrity, perseverance and courage among others were identified as consequential not only for the individual advanced practice nursing practitioner/aspirant but for the entire community of scholars/practitioners.

Person-centeredness was detailed and several models were explored and in particular the "five-dimension framework; 'biopsychosocial perspective'; 'person-as-person'; 'sharing power and responsibility'; 'therapeutic alliance'; and 'doctor-as-person'", by Mead and Bower (2000), each representing a particular aspect of the clinical encounter. In addition enablers, principles and activities based on the literature on patient-centered care were described. The essence of patient-centered care necessitates that the advanced practice nursing practitioner views the health care experience through the patient's eyes, rather than solely from a patient/client satisfaction experience survey.

Communities of Practice involve more than networking or exchanging data, for outreach to have an impact, the partnership needs to be reciprocal between the university and the community. This reciprocal cycle facilitated by advanced practice nursing practitioners can add to the knowledge base of nursing, while at the same time providing the community with valuable research-based information that can help formulate policy decisions that have long-term impact on citizens.

Communities of Practice align with the Scholarship of Engagement. The advanced practice nursing practitioner/aspirant would gain much in this scenario to progress meeting the criteria of clinical scholarship. The spectrum of clinical scholarship in Fig. 4.1 could be utilised as the model for the advanced practice nursing practitioner/aspirant to begin engaging with their portfolio in order to populate elements of the declared legacy/destination statement. Further, the advanced practice nursing practitioner/aspirant who enacts the scholarship of engagement through an ethic of a Community of Practice could raise the profile of person-centered care and embrace the deeper meaning of person-centeredness across a culture of care.

References

Barry M, Edgman-Levitan S. Shared decision making --- the pinnacle of patient-centered care. New Engl J Med. 2012;366:780–1.

Bell E, Campbell S, Goldberg L. Nursing identity and patient-centeredness in scholarly health services research: a computational text analysis of PubMed abstracts 1986-2013. BMC Health Serv Res. 2015;15:3. https://doi.org/10.1186/s12913-014-0660-8.

Benner P. From novice to expert. Menlo Park, CA: Addison-Wesley Publishing Company; 1984.

Benner P, Tanner C, Chesla C. Expertise in nursing practice. New York, NY: Springer Publishing Company; 1996.

Boyer E. Scholarship reconsidered: priorities of the professoriate. Carnegie Foundation for the Advancement of Teaching. Princeton, NJ: Princeton University Press; 1990.

Boyer E. The scholarship of engagement. J Publ Serv Outreach. 1996;1:11–20.

Boykin A, Schoenhofer S. Nursing as caring: a model for transforming practice. New York NY: National League for Nursing Press; 1993.

Brooker D. What is person centered care? Rev Clin Gerontol. 2004;13:215–22.

Brown M, Crabtree K. The development of practice scholarship in DNP programs: a paradigm shift. J Prof Nurs. 2013;29:330–7.

Brown J, Duguid P. The social life of information. Harvard Business School Press, Boston, MA,2000.

Bruns K, Conklin N, Wright M, Hoover D, Brace B, Wise G, Pendleton F, Dann M, Martin M, Childers J. Scholarship: the key to creating change through outreach. J High Educ Outreach Engag. 2003;8:3–11.

Bryant-Lukosious D, Martin-Misener R, Tranmer J, Donald F, Brousseau L, DiCenso A. Resources to facilitate advanced practice nursing outcome research. In: Kleinpell R, editor. Outcome assessment in advanced practice nursing. New York, NY: Springer Publishing Company; 2017. p. 250–71.

Cameron-Traub E. Clinical, conceptual and empirical aspects of nursing practice. In: Gray G, Pratt R, editors. Scholarship in the discipline of nursing. Melbourne, VIC: Churchill Livingstone; 1995. p. 1–20.

Carter E, Mastro K, Vose C, Rivera R, Larson E. Clarifying the conundrum: evidence-based practice, quality improvement or research? J Nurs Adm. 2017;47:266–70.

Chinchilla M, Arcaya M. Using health impact assessment as an interdisciplinary teaching tool. Int J Environ Teach Tool. 2017;14:744. https://doi.org/10.3390/ijerph14070744.

Clayman M, Pandit A, Bergeron A, Cameron K, Ross E, Wolf M. Ask, understand, remember: a brief measure of patient communication self-efficacy within clinical encounters. J Health Commun. 2010;15(Suppl):72–9.

Clissett P, Porock D, Hatwood R, Gladman J. The challenges of achieving person-centered care in acute hospitals: a qualitative study of people with dementia and their families. Int J Nurs Stud. 2013;50:1495–503.

Confessore S. Building a learning organisation: communities of practice. Self-directed learning and continuing medical education. J Contin Educ Health Prof. 1997;17:5–11.

Constand M, MacDermid J, Bello-Haas V, Law M. Scoping review of patient-centered care approaches in healthcare. BMC Health Serv Res. 2014;14:271.. Accessed from https://bmchealthservres.biomedcentral.com/articles/10.1186/1472-6963-14-271.

Cromarty I. What do patients think about during their consultations: a qualitative study. Br J Gen Pract. 1996;46:525–8.

Curry T, Naish J, Beacock C, Smith V. Real choice in the health service: an RCN discussion document. London: Royal College of Nursing; 2005.

Delaney L. Patient-centered care as an approach to improving health care in Australia. Collegian. 2018;25:119–23.

Diers D. Clinical scholarship. J Prof Nurs. 1995;11:24–30.

Diers D. Speaking of nursing narratives of practice, research, policy and profession. Burlington, MA: Jones and Bartlett Publishers; 2004.

Dopson S. A view from organisational studies. Nurs Res. 2007;56:572.

Edvardsson D, Fetherstonhaugh D, Nay R. Promoting a continuation of self and normality: person-centered care described by people with dementia, their family members and aged care staff. J Clin Nurs. 2010;19:2611–8.

Edwards C, Stanisezeswka S, Crichton N. Investigation of the ways in which patients reports of their satisfaction with healthcare are constructed. Sociol Health Illn. 2004;26:159–83.

Elwyn G, Frosch D, Thomson R, Joseph-Williams N, Lloyd A, Kinnersley P, Cordling E, Tomson D, Dodd C, Rollinick S, Edwards A, Barry M. Shared decision making: a model for clinical practice. J Gen Intern Med. 2012;27:1361–7.

Elwyn G, Coulter A, Laitner S, Walker E, Watson P, Thomson R. Implementing shared decision making in the NHS. BMJ. 2010;341:e5146.

Epstein R, Franks P, Fiscella K, Shields C, Meldrum S, Kravitz R, et al. Measuring patient-centered in patient-physician consultations: theoretical and practical issues. Soc Sci Med. 2005;61:1516–28.

Fear F, Rosaen C, Foster-Fishman P, Bawden R. Outreach as scholarly expression a faculty perspective. J High Educ Outreach Engag. 2001;6:21–34.

Fear F, Sandmann L. The "new" scholarship: implications for engagement and extension. J High Educ Outreach Engag. 2001–2002;7(1&2):29–39.

Ferguson-Pare M. What is a community of scholars in the practice environment? Nurs Sci Q. 2005;18:120. https://doi.org/10.1177/0894318405275863.

Gerteis M, Edgman-Levitan S, Daley J, Delbanco T. Through the patient's eyes. Jossey Bass: San Francisco, CA; 1993.

Glassick C, Huber M, Maeroff G. Scholarship assessed-evaluation of the professoriate. San Francisco, CA: Jossey-Bass; 1997.

Goodrich J, Cornwell J. Seeing the person in the patient: the point of carer review paper. London: King's Fund; 2008.

Greene S, Tuzzio L, Cherkin D. A framework for making patient-centered care front and center. Perm J. 2012;16:49–53.

Henwood F, Wyatt S, Hart A, Smith J. Ignorance is bliss sometimes: constraints on the emergence of the informed patient in the changing landscape of health information. Sociol Health Illn. 2003;25:589–607.

Hobbs J. A dimensional analysis of patient-centered care. Nurs Res. 2009;58:52–62.

Huber M. Teaching travels: reflections on the social life of classroom inquiry and innovation. Int J Scholar Teach Learn. 2009;3:1–7.

Hughes J, Bamford C, May C. Types of centeredness in health care: themes and concepts. Med Health Care Philos. 2008;11:455–63.

Institute of Medicine. Crossing the quality chasm: a new health system for the 21st Century. Washington, DC: National Academy Press; 2001.

Irvine D. Time for hard decisions on patient-centred professionalism. Med J Aust. 2004;181:271–4.

Ishikawa H, Hashimoto H, Kiuchi T. The evolving concept of "patient-centeredness" in patient-physician communication research. Soc Sci Med. 2013;96:147–53.

Jayadevappa R, Chhatre S. Patient centered care-a conceptual model and review of the state of the art. Open Health Serv Pol J. 2011;4:15–25.

Kitson A. The relevance of scholarship for nursing research and practice. J Adv Nurs. 2006;55:541–3.

Kitwood T. Dementia reconsidered: the person comes first. Bristol: Open University Press; 1997.

Kontos P, Naglie G. Bridging theory and practice: imagination, the body and person-centered dementia care. Dementia. 2007;6:549–69.

Kreindler S. The politics of patient-centred care. Health Expect. 2013;18:1139–50.

LeGrow K, Espin S. Beginning exploration of connectedness between patient-centered care, practice development and advanced nursing competencies to promote development. Int Pract Dev J. 2017;7:112. https://doi.org/10.19043/ipdj.72.008.

Leininger M. Leininger's theory of nursing: cultural care diversity and universality. Nurs Sci Q. 1988;1:152–60.

Little P, Everitt H, Williamson L, Warner G, Moore M, Gould C, Ferrier K, Payne S. Preferences of patents for patient-centered approach to consultation in primary care: an observational study. BMJ. 2001;322:468–72.

Lutz B, Bowers B. Patient-centered care: understanding its interpretation and implementation in health care. Sch Inq Nurs Pract. 2000;14:165–83.

Manley K, McCormack B. Person-centered care. Nurs Manage. 2008;15:12–3.

McCance T. Caring in nursing practice. The development of a conceptual framework. Res Theor Nurs Pract. 2003;17:101–16.

McCormack B, McCance T. Development of a framework for person-centred nursing. J Adv Nurs. 2006;56:472–9.

McCormack L, Treiman K, Rupert D, Williams-Piehota P, Nadler E, Arora N, et al. Measuring patient-centered communication in cancer care: a literature review and the development of a systematic approach. Soc Sci Med. 2011;72:1085–95.

McCormack B, McCance T, Maben J. Outcome evaluation in the development of person-centered practice. In: McCormack B, Manley K, Tichen A, editors. Practice development in nursing. Oxford: Wiley-Blackwell; 2013. p. 190–211.

McCormack B, McCance T. Person-centred practice in nursing and health care: theory and practice. 2nd ed. Chichester: Wiley Blackwell; 2017.

McCormack B, Borg M, Cardiff S, Dewing J, Jacobs G, Janes N, Karlsson B, McCance T, Mekki T, Porock D, Van Lieshout F, Wilson V. Person-centeredness – the state of the art. Int Pract Dev J. 2015;5(Suppl):1.. Accessed from https://www.fons.org/library/journal-ipdj-home.

McDermott R. Why information technology inspired but cannot deliver knowledge management. Calif Manage Rev. 1999;4:103–17.

McManus E, O'Connor L, Casey M. Health literacy and type 2 diabetes: Role of the pharmacist. Ir Pharm. 2017;12:33–6.

Mead N, Bower P. Patient-centeredness: a conceptual framework and review of the empirical literature. Soc Sci Med. 2000;51:1087–110.

Meehan T. Careful nursing: a model for contemporary nursing practice. J Adv Nurs. 2003;44:99–107.

Meleis A. On the way to scholarship: from master's to doctorate. J Prof Nurs. 1992;8:328–34.

Mercer S, Reynolds W. Empathy and quality care. Br J Gen Pract. 2002;52:S9–S12.

Mundinger M, Starck P, Hathaway D, Shaver J, Woods N. The ABCs of the doctor of nursing practice: assessing resources, building a culture of clinical scholarship, curricular models. J Prof Nurs. 2009;25:69–74.

Nightingale F. Notes on nursing. London: Appleton and Company; 1859.

Nightingale F. Florence Nightingale to Colonel Lloyd Lindsay. London: British Red Cross; 1882.

O'Connor, L. Developing 'subject matter experts': an important methodology program for acute postoperative pain with patients post major surgery. J Clin Nurs. 2016. https://doi.org/10.1111/jocn.13308.

O'Connor L, Casey M, Smith R, Fealy G, O'Brien D, O'Leary D, Stokes D, McNamara M, Glasgow ME, Cashin A. The universal, collaborative and dynamic model of specialist and advanced nursing and midwifery practice: a way forward? J Clin Nurs. 2018;27(5-6):e882–e894. https://doi.org/10.1111/jocn.13964.

Palmer I. The emergence of clinical scholarship as a professional imperative. J Prof Nurs. 1986;2:318–25.

Poland F, Birt L. The agentic person: shifting the focus of care. Aging Ment Health. 2016;20:771–2.

Pulvirenti M, McMillan J, Lawn S. Empowerment, patient centered care and self-management. Health Expect. 2014;17:303–10.

Pyrko I, Dorfler V, Eden C. Thinking together: what makes communities of practice work? Hum Relat. 2017;70:389–409.

Quatrara B, Dale Shaw K. Selecting advanced practice nursing outcomes measures. In: Kleinpell R, editor. Outcome assessment in advanced practice nursing. New York, NY: Springer Publishing Company; 2017. p. 45–58.

Quinn J, Smith M, Ritenbaugh C, Swanson K, Watson J. Research guidelines for assessing the impact of the healing relationship in clinical nursing. Altern Ther Health Med. 2003;9:A65–79.

Rathert C, Wyrwich M, Boren SA. Patient-centered care and outcomes: a systematic review of the literature. Med Care Res Rev. 2012;70:351–79.

Richards T, Coulter A, Wicks P. Time to deliver patient-centered care. BMJ. 2015;350: h530, 2018, https://doi.org/10.1136/BMJ.

Roach MS. The human act of caring: a blueprint for the health professions. Ottawa, NJ: Canadian Hospital Association; 1987.

Rolfe G. Nursing scholarship and the asymmetrical professor. Nurse Educ Pract. 2007;7:123–7.

Sakallaris B, Miller W, Saper R, Kreitzer M, Jonas W. Meeting the challenge of a more person-centered future for US healthcare. Global Adv Health Med. 2016;5:51–60. https://doi.org/10.7453/gahmj.2015-085.

Schlotfeldt R. Why promote clinical nursing scholarship? Clin Nurs Res. 1992;1:5–8.

Scott J, Cohen D, DiCicco-Bloom B, Miller W, Stange K, Crabtree B. Understanding healing relationships in primary care. Ann Fam Med. 2008;9:315–22.

Selden C, Zorn M, Ratzan S, Parker R. Health literacy. In: Current bibliographies in medicine. National Library of Medicine: Bethesda, MD; 2000.

Sherbino J, Snell L, Dath D, et al. A national clinician-educator program: a model of an effective community of practice. Med Educ Online. 2010;6:15.

STTI. Sigma Theta Tau International Clinical Scholarship resource paper. 1999. Accessed 17 December 2015, from http://www.nursingsociety.org/about-stti/position-statements-and-resource-papers.

Smith R. Making teaching count in Canadian higher education: developing a national agenda. Teaching and learning in higher education. Newsletter of the Society for Teaching and Learning in Higher Education (STLHE). Ottawa, ON: STLHE; 1997. p. 1–10.

Stewart M, Brown J, Weston W, McWhinney I, McWilliam C, Freeman T. Patient-centered medicine: transforming the clinical method. London: Sage; 1995.

Stewart M. The impact of patient-centered care on outcomes. J Fam Pract. 2000;49:796–804.

Stewart M. Towards a global definition of patient centered care. BMJ. 2001;322:444–5.

Stewart M, Brown J, Weston W, McWhinney I, McWilliam C, Freeman T. Patient-centered medicine: transforming the clinical method. 2nd ed. Oxford: Radcliffe, Medical Press; 2003.

Vistinainer M. The nature of knowledge and theory in nursing. Image. 1986;18:32–7.

Wenger E. Communities of practice: learning, meaning and identity. Cambridge: Cambridge University Press; 1998.

World Health Organisation (WHO). Health promotion Ottawa charter for health promotion. WHO, Geneva; 1986.

World Health Organisation. Global strategy on people-centered and integrated health care services. Geneva: World Health Organisation; 2015.

Wilkies L, Mannix J, Jackson D. Practicing nurses perspectives of clinical scholarship: a qualitative study. BMC Nurs. 2013;12:21. Accessed from https://bmcnurs.biomedcentral.com/articles/10.1186/1472-6955-12-21.

Zill J, Scholl I, Harter M, Dirmaler J. Which dimensions of patient-centeredness matter? Results of a web-based expert Delphi survey. PLoS One. 2015;10:e0141978. https://doi.org/10.1371/journal.pone.0141978.

Doctorate of Nursing Practice: A Conduit for Scholarship in the Realm of Advanced Practice

5

5.1 Introduction

This chapter explores the doctor of nursing practice and Boyer's dimensions of scholarship. Engaging in the scholarship of practice is unraveled and its relationship with advanced practice nursing professional education. The entry pathway to advanced practice nursing is presented in light of the literature and various pipelines associated with entry into advanced practice. Some debate abounds pertinent to the doctor of nursing practice and doctor of philosophy especially in the context of an advanced practice career pathway. The evolutions of the various modes of knowledge production are discussed in the milieu of the doctor of nursing practice. Scholarship as a conduit in the realm of advanced practice nursing is interwoven in the text and the challenges therein. The potential opportunities for advanced practice nursing practitioners to become a knowledge broker is recommended for inclusion in future scholarly conversations.

5.2 Doctoral and Professional Education for Advanced Practice Links to Boyer's Model

The ideas expressed by Boyer (1990) in *Scholarship Reconsidered* and other powerful trends affecting doctoral and professional education have led to explicit recognition that students in advanced degree programs will face diverse and challenging career options, and responsibilities and thus need to develop an array of abilities, competencies and capabilities. In addition to developing deep knowledge in one's discipline, these competences, attitudes, and abilities, echoing emphases found in *Scholarship Reconsidered*, include an understanding that scholarly talents may take many forms. These talents include the ability to share and connect one's expertise with that of others in order to apply knowledge in service to solving problems, skills in assessing one's own work and that of others, an attitude of flexibility, and a

© Springer Nature Switzerland AG 2019
L. O'Connor, *The Nature of Scholarship, a Career Legacy Map and Advanced Practice*, Advanced Practice in Nursing, https://doi.org/10.1007/978-3-319-91695-8_5

commitment to on-going learning (Austin and McDaniels 2016). Doctoral and professional programs, as well as national organisations and associations, are developing new ways to help future academics and professionals develop this array of skills and capabilities that will mark them as scholars and professionals needed in today's challenging and changing academic and professional settings (NMBI 2017; DoH 2017; Austin and McDaniels 2016).

All forms of scholarship require a broad intellectual foundation. Tomorrow's scholars must be liberally educated and must think creatively, communicate effectively, and have the capacity and the inclination to place ideas in a larger context (Boyer 1990, p. 65). At the outset most students should continue to pursue a specialised field of study and do original research. However, all students increasingly should be encouraged to work across the specialities, taking courses in other disciplines to gain a broader perspective (Boyer 1990, p. 68). The point is that even as the categories of human knowledge have become more and more discreet, the need for transdisciplinary insight has increased. Indeed, the tangible risk is that graduate students will become specialists without perspective, that they will have technical competence but lack larger insights. Therefore, to avoid such narrowness an integrative component should be built into every program (Boyer 1990, p. 68). Specifically, all doctoral candidates should be urged to put their special area of study in historical perspective and that time during graduate study also should be devoted to social and ethical concerns, so that the scholar finds metaphors and paradigms that give larger meaning to specialised knowledge (Boyer 1990).

Within this context of critique and reform in doctoral and professional education, several themes of Boyer's work have been particularly pertinent to such discussions and developments. First, scholarly work takes a variety of forms. Boyer suggested a broader view of scholarship that includes teaching, integration, application, engagement as well as discovery. Specifically, when scholarship is recognised to take several overlapping yet interdependent forms, the preparation of advanced practice nursing practitioners with an ability to engage in Boyer's domains of scholarship within their discipline and related speciality requires the development of capability in several areas. These areas include, mastering foundational knowledge; developing skills to advance knowledge in nursing; understanding the importance of the integration and the relationships among bodies of knowledge across various specialities. Finally, knowing how to apply knowledge to problems of practice within one's speciality or in a transdisciplinary context and in national, and international communities is essential while demonstrating effective approaches to disseminating that knowledge so that it impacts on practice (Austin and McDaniels 2016).

That said, all forms of scholarship benefit from documentation, peer, public and self-scrutiny. In fact, part of scholarship is the activity of evaluating and learning from self and with others. Thus scholars should document their professional practice and participate actively in assessment processes of their own work along with the work of others and complete a portfolio legacy map (see Chap. 6). Evaluation processes should take into account and respect all forms of scholarship including engagement, discovery, integration, application, and teaching incorporating the six standards of evaluation outlined by Glassick et al. (1997). It is these complex challenges that call for the preparation of a new generation of scholars, "triple-helix"

(Thune 2010), who are prepared for dynamic roles across a variety of contexts. Traditionally, the term *scholar* has been used to describe individuals who have terminal research degrees, are experts in their disciplines, and enjoy engaging in scholarly activities where ideas and knowledge are currency. Such individuals are prepared and certified by doctoral programs to engage in work that may but not limited to, research problem identification, utilization of existing literature to situate research questions, project design and implementation, collection and analysis of data, and the communication of research results to various audiences (McDaniels and Skogsberg 2017). Moreover, Boyer (1990) recommended that the scholarship of engagement, application, discovery, integration and teaching should be part of the education vernacular for all students.

5.3 Doctor of Nursing Practice: Scholarship Revisited

Growth in education and practice for advanced practice in nursing is occurring in tandem with a confused scope of practice, the need for health care cost containment, fragmented educational and training criteria, and qualifications leading to challenging health care delivery (Schober and Affara 2006). The Department of Health (2017) draft policy presented a framework for graduate, specialist and advanced nursing and midwifery practice in Ireland capable of developing a critical mass of nurses and midwives to address emerging and future service needs, including driving integration between acute and community services (DoH 2017). In most countries, including Ireland, a master's degree in nursing is now recommended or required for qualification as an advanced practice nursing practitioner/nurse practitioner (NCNZ 2017; Parker and Hill 2017). Preparation for advanced nursing practice in the United States is at doctoral level since 1979 (Parker and Hill 2017; Koskinen et al. 2012; ANA 2010) and at master's level in Australia (ANMAC 2015). In Australia, advanced practice nursing and advanced practice roles have been conceptualised through application of the Strong Model (Gardner et al. 2013, 2016).

Entry into advanced practice nursing programs in the USA has been visualised as a pipeline (Deatrick 2011), that comes in various sizes with different input and output filters (Danaher Hacker et al. 2015). Unfortunately, attempts to streamline entry into advanced practice nursing such as doctor of nursing practice (DNP) degree, have resulted in unintended consequences that may end up strangling the pipeline and putting undue financial pressure on institutions that have chosen to solely move forward with DNP programs (Danaher Hacker et al. 2015). Meanwhile, Martsolf et al. (2015) reported that the transition to the DNP degree has not been universally accepted in the USA, resulting in multiple lengths for the pipeline into advanced practice nursing, while according to Danaher Hacker et al. (2015) market forces may prevail rather than the "collective genius" of our [nursing] profession (p. 386).

It should be emphasised according to Dreher (2011) that the doctor of nursing practice (DNP) degree was not created because the Masters was becoming inferior or because master's-prepared advanced practice nurses have poor outcomes. On the contrary, Mundinger et al. (2000) found primary care outcomes to be the same when comparing nurse practitioners (with master's degrees) to physicians, while a systematic review by Horrocks et al. (2002) found no differences in prescriptions, return consultations, or referrals between nurse practitioners' care and physicians in primary care settings. Moreover, positive findings reported by Ellis (2006) indicated that the professional doctorate created informed nurses who viewed themselves as being '*equal to medical staff*', and empowered to make changes (Ellis 2006, p. 489).

Kot and Hendel (2012) note that the development of the professional doctorate in Australia is linked not only to criticisms of the traditional PhD but to factors such as employability of holders of doctoral degrees, the growth of the knowledge economy and the changing role of higher education and government involvement. Earlier work by Ellis (2006) using a modified form of illuminative evaluation was to present as full and complete account of the Australian professional doctorates for nurses to inform the development of the professional doctorate within the UK and elsewhere by: (1) conducting a reconnaissance and detailed mapping of the Australian professional doctorates for nurses to identify the characteristics and features of such programmes; (2) obtaining the views of some key stakeholders on the professional doctorate for nurses; and (3) identifying the similarities and differences between the PhD and the professional doctorate (Ellis 2006). Data were obtained from students enrolled on one of the professional doctorates (n = 14) in Australia. Participants were interviewed on a one-to-one basis. Respondents worked in a range of settings including mental health; operating theatres; emergency nursing; acute care; transplant services; and oncology and two of the participants were lecturers. Most, but not all of the students were senior practitioners with between 5 and 15 years clinical experience in their specialist field (Ellis 2006). The findings suggest students saw little point in pursuing research that was unrelated to their practice and viewed the PhD as belonging to the realm of academia; *"I really wanted to be seen not as an academic with a research degree but as a clinical leader with a research degree, with academic degrees (the PhD) they have no idea about clinical practice"* (Year 3) (Ellis 2006, p. 488).

Nurses have generally not seen the PhD as the best fit for their higher professional development. Accordingly, the professional doctorate offers a compelling and dynamic alternative to the more academic focus of the PhD and prepares 'inquiry-driven leaders' for tomorrow's challenges (Walker et al. 2016, p. 60). Rolfe and Davies (2009) make two main points in respect of the development of the professional doctorate: professional doctorates have arisen out of dissatisfaction with the traditional PhD which is perceived as too distant from practice; and study at doctoral level is now increasingly relevant to those working outside academe.

Pearson (1999) noted 20 years ago, the continuing debate about the status of professional doctorates demonstrates how the view of the traditional PhD is embedded as primarily an individual student's research project and how fundamentally conservative the response to change has been despite the extent of innovative initiatives. Besides, Heasling (1986) described the PhD, for example, as 'a traditional credential attribute of an individual awarded by an institute of higher education after successful defence of a dissertation, recording the candidate's independent and original contribution to knowledge'. The PhD then, is clearly and not problematically, the degree of choice for someone seeking a career in the academy or as a professional researcher (Walker et al. 2016).

Meanwhile, the professional doctorate enables staff to become what Bourner et al. (2001) have called 'researching professionals' as opposed to 'professional researchers' or correspondingly, Gregory's (1997) view of 'scholarly professionals' vis-à-vis 'professional scholars'. The professional researcher/scholar, due to the nature and scope of the traditional dissertation, should produce knowledge that is more theoretical or generate more evidence-based practice knowledge when working with larger data sets with an emphasis on heterogeneity of samples and the generalisability of findings (Dreher 2011). On the other hand, the professional doctorate is a combination of rigorous coursework and a major piece of research and together these activities have the express aim of producing what Walker et al. (2016) have also called 'researching professionals' as opposed to professional researchers. This distinction according to Walker et al. (2016) is important insofar as it recognises the primary aim of the professional doctorate is to improve healthcare through the actions of the researchers undertaking their doctorate. A PhD can, but does not usually, have such an emphasis on the context *in situ* of healthcare and the systems and processes required to deliver that health care to the very highest standards possible. The professional doctorally prepared nurse, however, is able to do exactly that (Walker et al. 2016, p. 67).

Stew (2009) emphasised that the professional doctorate graduate is expected to be an "advanced practitioner rather than a career researcher" (p. 1). However, Dreher (2011) questions whether the advanced practice nurse can be properly educated to engage in real advanced practice if they complete a professional doctorate that excluded new experiences or the establishment of new practice competencies beyond the master's degree. The term doctoral advanced nursing practice (or doctoral advanced practice nursing) may actually provide more clarity and better differentiate the skill set of an advanced practice nurse with a doctorate from an advanced practice nurse with a master's degree (Dreher and Montgomery 2009). What is unknown, however, is whether the healthcare market will widely embrace a doctoral practitioner with enhanced competencies or ultimately, whether a critical mass of these nursing graduates can improve health (Dreher 2011, p. 405). According to Barkham et al. (2010) in relation to the professional doctorate that the concept of practice-based evidence "… provides the foundations for generating research questions that are grounded in the practice context and, for this reason, need to be relevant to practitioners and the delivery of routine services" (p. 41).

The American Association of Colleges of Nursing recommended that schools of nursing transition their advanced practice registered nurse (APRN) programs to doctor of nursing practice (DNP) programs by 2015. In October 2004, the American Association of Colleges of Nursing (AACN) adopted a position statement affirming the role and development for *practice* doctorates in nursing:

"the practice-focused doctoral program will be a distinct model of doctoral education that provides an additional option for attaining a terminal degree in the discipline" (AACN p. 8). The document states that there will be perceived benefits of such a degree that include notions of enhanced knowledge to improve nursing

practice and patient outcomes. Doctoral programs in nursing and other applied scientific disciplines have been categorised into two distinct types: research-focused and practice-focused. The AACN (2004) defined the term *practice* to include:

> *any form of nursing intervention that influences healthcare outcomes for individuals or populations, including the direct care of individual patients, management and care for individuals and populations, administration of nursing and healthcare organisations, and the development of health care policy. Preparation at the practice doctorate level includes advanced preparation in nursing based on nursing science, and is at the highest level of nursing practice (p. 3).*

Besides, McVicar et al. (2006) offered some valuable defining evidence criteria of the professional doctorate as follows:

- The research focus is 'the solution of problems in practice and the generation of new knowledge to inform improvements in practice' (Galvin and Carr 2003). Notably this criterion recognises 'practice as scholarship' (Ramcharan et al. 2001; Newman 1997; Pearson et al. 1997);
- It is interventionist in relationship to the subject being investigated; and
- It embraces an applied, problem-focused, or action-based approach to proposing or implementing change in the organisations in which the student is involved (McVicar et al. 2006).

The authors further state that while these features could likewise appear in a PhD, the difference between the PhD and professional doctorate is that the focus on addressing the needs of the student's own organisation is the critical factor (McVicar et al. 2006). In addition, Bourner et al. (2001) note that a student undertaking the professional doctorate commences the research from an understanding of their practice, leading to an identification of a problem for investigation, and finishes by applying their learning in resolving the issue. Furthermore, McVicar et al. (2006) state that although the professional doctorate commences from a different position to that of a PhD, the end-point in terms of the critical benchmarks observed in doctoral theses are similar, including originality, depth of analysis and level of synthesis. Similarly, there is an expectation that students will publish their findings. Trafford and Lesham (2002a, b) echo these views by proposing that while their design may differ, the PhD and professional doctorate should share similarities that characterise scholarship, enquiry and externally verified standards, and ultimately lead to an original contribution either by filling a gap in, or by extending knowledge (McVicar et al. 2006). A cross-sectional study conducted in the USA aimed to identify barriers and facilitators to academic careers for doctor of nursing practice (DNP) students. One thousand five hundred DNP students were randomly selected from nursing schools across the country to participate in the survey, and a 56.9% response rate was achieved (Fang and Bednash 2017). Given that research is not a focus of DNP education in the USA, the finding that more than 60% of students who planned to pursue an academic career felt confident in conducting independent research was reported as interesting (Fang and Bednash 2017). Because the term *independent research* was not defined in the survey, students may have interpreted it freely. However, the finding that only 32.5% of the same students felt confident in writing research proposals, which is a necessary skill for research that are hypothesis driven and require scientific methodology, suggests that a large majority of these students may not be prepared for independent research (Fang and Bednash 2017).

5.4   Evolution from First to Second to Third Generation Professional Doctorates

The first professional doctorates in Australia and elsewhere, referred to as first generation professional doctorates (Maxwell 2003), were only structurally dissimilar from the PhD insofar as they typically consisted of course work followed by a thesis and were dominated by academe (Maxwell and Shanahan 1997). The equivalent was also said to relate to those in the United Kingdom, generally referred to as 'taught doctorates' which are typically a blend of taught modules that must be passed, followed by a research study which may be applied and clinically based (Park 2007).

Several researchers (Maxwell 2011; Rolfe and Davies 2009; Wallgren and Dahlgren 2005) have progressed the work of Gibbons et al. (1994) as a very useful taxonomy of knowledge-production in distinguishing the epistemological contours that differentiate the PhD (Mode 1) from the professional doctorate (Mode 2). In Mode 1 (PhD), knowledge development by tradition is that problems arise, are tested, then analysed within very accepted paradigms, and subsequently published in peer reviewed journals and disseminated (Gibbons et al. 1994). The *generation* of knowledge through research is kept separate from and uncontaminated by the *application* of that knowledge to practice, on the assumption that 'discovery must precede application' (Gibbons et al. 1994, p. 33). Meanwhile, Mode 2 knowledge generation, is based within the workplace, is context-driven, heterogeneous in terms of the skills and experience people bring to it, transdisciplinary, and has an outcome that may take many different forms (Gibbons et al. 1994, p. 6). A key feature of Mode 2 is transdisciplinary, that is, the ability to work outside of academe and solve problems in context; hence its appeal to advanced practice nursing practitioners who wish to change or improve practice in their own workplace (Rolfe and Davies 2009). Of note, Gibbons et al. (1994) describes their concept of transdisciplinary in the context of Mode 2 knowledge production:

"The transdisciplinary mode of knowledge production described by us does not necessarily aim to establish itself as a new, transdisciplinary discipline, nor is it inspired by restoring cognitive unity. On the contrary, it is essentially a temporary configuration and thus highly mutable. It takes its particular shape and generates the content of its theoretical and methodological core in response to problem-formulations that occur in highly specific and local contexts of application" (Gibbons et al. 1994, pp. 29–30). According to Rolfe and Davies (2009) the idea of a transdisciplinary curriculum of the type advocated by Gibbons et al. for Mode 2 knowledge-production extends a great deal further than merely a reorganisation of

existing disciplinary boundaries and power relationships '... transdisciplinary entails not only transcendence of disciplinary boundaries, but to some extent the transcendence of the *very idea* of disciplines' (p. 1270).

Walker et al. (2016) argue the 'traditional' PhD is more marked by Mode 1 knowledge-production than the professional doctorate, which conversely, derives its epistemological (as well as socio-political) capital from Mode 2 knowledge-production. Within Gibbons' et al. (1994) taxonomy, Rolfe and Davies (2009) explain that the traditional Mode 1 PhD is usually situated within a single and discrete academic discipline, such that the boundaries of relevant knowledge and theory, along with the valid and accepted methods for generating and disseminating that knowledge, are secure and largely uncontested (pp. 1267–1268). Furthermore, Mode 1 knowledge production is 'driven by an academic agenda, categorised by the associated disciplines ... residing in the University, where they are guarded by an academic elite'. Besides, under this Mode 1 knowledge production 'students are inducted into the disciplinary knowledge and practice of the University and to be successful they must align themselves to the theoretical and methodological frameworks which characterise these' (Rolfe and Davies 2009, pp. 1267–1268). Therefore, based on the these explanations, it could be interpreted that the PhD is a product of and for the University rather than any other place; a point reinforced by Maxwell and Kupczyck-Romanczuk (2009) who acknowledged that the focus of professional doctorate work is the community of practice, as opposed to the community of academics. Another detail outlined by Rolfe and Davies that warrants noting'. ...at the outset the focus of Gibbons' et al. distinction between Mode 1 and Mode 2 is on *production* rather than *product*. Knowledge is categorised and valued according to how it is produced rather than what it looks like, and it therefore makes no sense to refer to Mode 1 or Mode 2 *knowledge* per se' (Rolfe and Davies 2009, p. 1267).

Mode 2 knowledge production is characterised by Gibbons et al. (1994) as:

'a constant flow back and forth between the fundamental and the applied, between the theoretical and the practical. Typically, discovery occurs in contexts where knowledge is developed for and put to use, while results—which would have been traditionally characterised as applied—fuel further theoretical advances' (p. 19). It is important to note according to Rolfe and Davies (2009) that Mode 2 represents an alternative to Mode 1 knowledge-production rather than a replacement and in this sense it complements the desire by universities to provide professional doctorates whilst preserving the traditional PhD. Mode 2 knowledge production has five characteristic elements, recognising that:

1. Knowledge is not produced separately to the context in which it is used
2. The range of sites where knowledge is produced is diverse
3. Knowledge is transdisciplinary and resides within individual practitioners and teams
4. Knowledge is reflexive and embedded, coming from somewhere as opposed to existing by itself ready to be discovered
5. Novel forms of quality control are indicated (Nowotny et al. 2005).

According to Lester (2004) second generation professional doctorates appear to be more accepting of Mode 2 knowledge-production 'being more equally rooted in the contexts of the academy, the profession and the work place or practicum' (p. 758). Under Mode 2, the link between theory and practice is more apparent as they become two sides of the same coin, and because research takes place in the workplace, knowledge-production and diffusion are interlinked (Rolfe and Davies 2009, p. 1268).

It has been identified that there is a marked paucity of published evidence of the impact of professional doctorates on patient care, or even of the impact of learning outcomes achievement on practitioners and students in nursing and across health-care disciplines (Ketefian and Redman 2015; Wilkies et al. 2013; Clearly et al. 2011; Watson et al. 2011; Reed 2006). This deficit applies not only in healthcare but in other professions (Kumar 2014). It is uncertain if this is exclusively the result of the noticeable lack of research, or if it reflects a lack of clarity in the design of professional doctorates that flows into difficulty in identification of researchable questions (Cashin et al. 2017). Therefore, an academic conversation needs to start about the future direction of doctoral education globally for advanced practice nursing. According to Thompson and Schwartz Barcott (2019) the knowledge broker role needs to be integrated into advanced practice curricular (i.e., doctoral studies) to teach the necessary skills and provide experiential learning. Knowledge brokering would enable the advanced practice nursing practitioner change the availability and access to information, improve health literacy and be responsive to underserved population needs, particularly in the context of social justice and empowerment (WHO 2004; O'Fallon et al. 2003). Being at the margin, advanced practice nursing practitioners can appreciate not only the system as a whole but also the needs of those located on the periphery and in that context working within marginality the advanced practice nursing practitioner can support social justice (Delvin et al. 2018, p. 114).

A systematic literature review by Hawkes and Yerrabati (2018) draws on the evidence of 193 academic papers to map out the existing academic knowledge about professional doctorates and highlights the gaps that warrant research. The findings reveal that literature is largely dominated by papers based in three countries: the USA (44%), the UK (31%) and Australia (17%). Very little has been written outside these three countries, and these are the same three countries in which professional doctorates are most dominant (Hawkes and Yerrabati 2018). Further, this systematic review highlights the need for academic work in this area to move beyond individual case studies of practice on programmes towards developing principles of practice for professional doctorates as a whole (Hawkes and Yerrabati 2018). The authors report that the literature on doctorates in education has led to general consensus on two important aspects—curriculum and student experience—the literature on other types of professional doctorates is limited (doctor in nursing = 13 papers out of 193) and there is therefore scope for research in these areas for other professional doctorates (Hawkes and Yerrabati 2018). Of note, the prime driver for the professional doctorate in education appeared to be industry related, or what Brennan refers to as "the production of useful knowledge to provide Australia with economic advantage" (Brennan 1995,

p. 22). Conversely, such an imperative is all too apparent within health care with an ageing population, the mounting costs of technology and the concomitant rise in consumer expectations (Ellis 2007). Further, Hawkes and Yerrabati (2018) identify two significant gaps in knowledge, even on the doctorates in education programmes. The first is literature on the wider impact of professional doctorates. While it is clear for those who work with professional doctoral students that there is a wider value, this is not well documented in the literature. The second is a significant gap in the taught aspects of the doctorate in education programme and little about the thesis stage and the role of the supervisor (Hawkes and Yerrabati 2018).

The emphasis on practice improvement drives the curricular content in DNP programs and requires that students possess a command of practice problems and the ability to access and assess evidence-based literature for solutions to practice problems (Brown and Crabtree 2013). The focus of the DNP practice was not viewed from the lens of discovery, but from a lens of translation of the "best" evidence into practice. The PhD was established to generate evidence, whereas the DNP role is to translate and disseminate evidence into practice. The continuous loop or life cycle of evidence translation not only impacts patient care at the point of delivery, but also is a stimulus for future research and discovery through measurable system-based improvement (Kirk Walker and Polancich 2015, p. 268).

Healthcare today and into the future is increasingly more complex and requires ever more highly skilled healthcare professionals to meet the challenges of providing safe, and evidenced-based quality care. Doctoral research and education based in the workplace and designed to improve healthcare while skilling up nurses and other professionals in research methods has never been more relevant and appropriate (Walker et al. 2016). The goal of doctor of nursing practice (DNP) programs should be to produce nurses that are uniquely prepared to bridge the gap between the discovery of new knowledge and the scholarship of translation, application, and integration of this new knowledge in practice (American Association of Colleges of Nursing [AACN], 2006). Knowledge generation is necessary—but not sufficient—to transform the role of nursing and lead change (Dreher et al. 2014). Nursing knowledge eventually must reach the public domain, where people and families personally feel its benefits. The DNP is the profession's best chance to increase the number of advanced practice nurses needed for health care transformation (Dreher et al. 2014). Doubling the number of nurses with a doctorate and removing the scope of practice barriers, alone, will not be sufficient to transform advanced practice education or the health care system. According to Dreher et al. (2014) there is an obligation to create not just curricula for advanced practice but *learning environments* in which nurse scientists and clinicians, working collaboratively, are joined by experts from other professions and disciplines to offer learning opportunities and experiences that will serve our students well—not just in 2020, but in 2030 and 2040 and 2050 (p. 108). The discipline of nursing has much to gain from embracing, rather than retreating from, the challenges posed by second generation professional doctorates, and these offer an alternative but no less academically sound education in preparing nurses to play a full and active role at the theory-practice interface (Rolfe and Davies 2009).

A scoping review of peer-reviewed literature in databases; CINAHL, Medline and PsycINFO from January 2000 until 2017 was undertaken by Cashin et al. (2017) pertinent to the development of professional doctorates in the discipline of nursing. The purpose of the review was to inform thinking with regard to future design work for a post-masters (nurse practitioner endorsement) professional doctorate (Cashin et al. 2017). The authors postulate that the discussion now needs to progress from second- to third-generation professional doctorates in nursing and move beyond the comparison with the PhD, to a discussion of a learning *product* at doctoral level that has internal coherence, and where course philosophy, learning outcomes, teaching and learning activity and assessment are clearly articulated. The learning product would not be judged against the PhD but rather against university (and societal) standards of doctoral education (Cashin et al. 2017). The doctorate degree would concentrate on building practice capability rather than producing nurse scientist capability. Accordingly, clear articulation of the learning *product* may indeed enable identification of findings that could begin a body of research that ascertains the impact of the doctorate on learners and also on the systems in which they practice at an advanced level. Such research is much needed to gauge the transformative nature and social robustness of the professional doctorate and to establish its place in development of nursing practice scholarship (Cashin et al. 2017).

5.5   Engaging in the Scholarship of Practice

Although informed by research, nursing is ultimately a practice discipline. The tension between the discipline and the profession and the role of the researcher-educator and the role of the practitioner-educator has pre-empted a more important and robust discussion in the USA of how research and practice complement each other (Dreher et al. 2014). Therefore, the most important question is how opportunities are created for both kinds of doctoral students, (PhD and DNP) to learn together, respect each other, and deploy their mutual strengths to form networks of practice and education models (Ketefian and Redman 2015; Dreher et al. 2014). Elevating advanced practice education to doctoral preparation allows for the identification of gaps in care and subsequent operationalising of translational research skills focused on improving clinical outcomes and quality care. Knowledge translation forms part of the knowledge-to-action cycle (Graham et al. 2006). The knowledge-to-action cycle details the sequence and steps involved in achieving the transfer of research knowledge into clinical practice consisting of a creation phase and an action phase (Curtis et al. 2016). Academic institutions will need to utilise continuous self-assessment metrics and outcomes of DNP education programs to ensure quality of care to the public as the profession embarks on etching nursing's newest doctorate into professional history (Paplham and Austin-Ketch 2015). A descriptive quality improvement project was conducted to evaluate the scholarly projects (n = 80) of Doctor of Nursing Practice education on one programme in the USA across four graduating classes using a modification of the Uncertainty, Pace, Complexity Model (Terhaar and Sylvia 2015). The aim of the investigation was to evaluate, monitor and manage the quality of projects conducted and work produced as evidence of scholarship upon completion of Doctor of Nursing Practice education. The level of scholarship and quality of work products matters to the future of the DNP degree and to the practice of nursing. It is critical therefore, that doctoral study produce doctoral level work; that such work can easily be distinguished from masters' level work and that the scholarship produced be original, impactful and practice-based (Terhaar and Sylvia 2015, p. 172). Analysis revealed that projects were well aligned with the strategic plan of the host organisation, focused directly on patient populations and accomplish the work of translation (Terhaar and Sylvia 2015).

The DNP has potential to improve clinical, operational and financial outcomes. Population demographics require it, complexity of health care delivery demands it, success of health care reform depends on it and the pressure to realise meaningful quality improvement will fail without it (Terhaar and Sylvia 2015). The conduct of rigorous, high quality, clinical projects that deliver improved outcomes will prepare DNPs to lead boundary-spanning quality improvement and translation activities across systems that can achieve the full potential of this practice doctorate (Terhaar and Sylvia 2015). The AACN Task Force proposed that while new knowledge gained from DNP scholarship activities may be transferable, it should not be considered generalizable, as is knowledge yielded from the traditional research doctorate, yet translational research also has value in the larger healthcare environment. The need for advanced practice nurses who are able to translate and apply research to the clinical setting is emphasised in the AACN Task Force report, which states that differences in knowledge generation, between practice and research-based doctorates, should not be viewed in a hierarchical relationship (AACN 2015). However, to ensure the greatest impact, DNP faculty should work closely with students to identify the setting that is the best match for the project population and outcomes (Alexander 2016). Earlier, Redman et al. (2015) conducted a database search for publications between 2005 and 2012 having at least one DNP-prepared author in attempts to determine DNP nurse productivity. The authors used publishing in areas of speciality or relevance to the DNP graduate as an indirect measure of leadership and demonstration of scholarship. Eight focus areas among 690 published articles were noted, including role of DNP; nursing education; clinical practice; health delivery systems/quality and safety; policy, administration, business, and executive; ethics; and other (Redman et al. 2015). Based on review of the publications, DNPs are engaged in strategic roles in practice and education and have cultivated writing scholarship, consistent with the intended outcomes of the AACN DNP *Essentials*. Redman et al. (2015) validate the need to document outcomes of DNP graduates, particularly measurement of the impact of translation of evidence to practice, ability to lead system and policy changes, and ultimately improvement in health care.

Compelling awareness, inspiring application, and engaging in the scholarship of practice has the potential to empower students to utilize empirical and/or theoretical evidence instead of relying upon "common sense" or "management fads" (Birnbaum 2000), as they enact professional practices while in their graduate training programs and over the course of their careers. It is also true that this process will be uncomfortable for some; it will require doctoral students to embrace a novice identity as they learn about the scholarship that exists on their work practices while at the same time strengthening their identities as experts (McDaniels and Skogsberg 2017, p. 80).

In the current economic climate and health care environment, advanced practice registered nurses (APRNs) need to be knowledgeable about the interpretation of cost, and effectiveness data in particular, when they are combined in a cost-effectiveness study (Bryant-Lukosius et al. 2015; Martin-Misener et al. 2015). To accomplish these goals, APRNs must understand how to distinguish comparative-effectiveness research from cost-effectiveness analysis (CEA) research and business case analyses (Frick et al. 2017). Comparative-effectiveness research is defined as the conduct and synthesis of research comparing the benefits and harms of diverse interventions and strategies to prevent, diagnose, treat, and monitor health conditions in "real-world" settings; its purpose is to improve health outcomes by developing and disseminating information about the everyday effectiveness of interventions (Volpp and Das 2009). This methodology is very much *patient-centered* and thus is also called *patient-centered outcome research*. This methodology not only highlights the everyday needs of the patients, but it may also incorporate many different types of patient outcomes (Frick et al. 2017, p. 21) and in addition identify the advanced practice nursing practitioners' contribution to the patient-centered agenda.

The current health care climate calls for attention to outcome measures. The advanced practice nursing practitioner will need to generate evidence of how nursing contributes to high-quality care and health service performance by developing a schema of quality and performance metrics that will track daily activities and align these to "what matters most to patients as individuals" (O'Connor et al. 2018, p. e891). Strategies that can be used to measure advanced practice nursing practitioner impact include establishing role-specific metrics, planning for outcome evaluation when any new role is established, and building in outcomes as a part of an institution's overall strategic plan to identify impact of the APRN role (Kapu et al. 2017). Furthermore, performance measures are often benchmarked or compared with other institutions. Benchmarking is a process to identify best practices, which, when implemented, can lead to superior performance (DesHarnais 2013). Further, data of performance measures are compared between health care systems or within a single health care system (DesHarnais 2013). These comparisons allow advanced practice nursing practitioners identify areas of strengths and weakness in relation to best practice (Gawlinski et al. 2017). In these instances the DNP program can build the scholarship conduit within the realm of clinical practice.

By virtue of their graduate education preparation, clinical knowledge, and critical thinking skills, APRNs have an essential role in evaluating outcomes for improvement efforts (Gawlinski et al. 2017). Yet, well-controlled studies on advanced practice registered nurses (APRN) outcomes continue to be relatively scant (Bryant-Lukosius et al. 2015; Stanik-Hutt et al. 2013; Newhouse et al. 2011). However, some do exist and suggest that APRNs "provide safe, effective, quality care to a number of specific populations in a variety of settings" (Stanik-Hutt et al. 2013; Newhouse et al. 2011). Advanced practice nursing practitioners are essential to the quality system initiatives that occur in clinical care settings. Their work directly influences patient care outcomes, consumer satisfaction, system efficiencies, and cost savings, but too often it is not recognised because it is "invisible". Though system outcomes may be hard to ascribe to any one individual, the contributions of APRNs are more likely to be acknowledged if data are available (Quatrara and Dale Shaw 2017).

In order to establish the effectiveness of a critical mass of advanced practice nursing practitioners', the dose of the intervention being delivered could be established which reflects their activities. Reed et al. (2007) outlined a protocol for measuring the dose of nursing interventions that allows for effectiveness of the intervention to be calculated. The dose is comprised of three key components, 1) amount, 2) frequency, and 3) duration of the intervention (Reed et al. 2007). The three components allow for the calculation of a *use rate* that can be analysed further (Reed et al. 2007). By establishing the dose, the impact of the critical mass of advanced practice nursing practitioners on relevant key performance indicators, such as patient waiting times, duration of consultations and treatments, return visits, care delivery in the appropriate setting, and unscheduled care visits can be determined. Hence, this activity data can become part of the data set to inform an economic evaluation of the role of the advanced practice nursing practitioner globally.

Udlis and Mancuso (2015) explored how nurses perceive the role of the DNP-prepared nurse and identified areas of ambiguity in understanding the roles that DNP-prepared nurses fulfil. A descriptive, cross-sectional design, using self-administered questionnaires, explored the perceptions of n = 340 nurses with various educational levels and backgrounds.

A majority of participants agreed that DNP-prepared nurses are able to help bridge the gap between science and practice (88%) and substantially contribute to nursing scholarship (63%). Furthermore, 57% of participants agreed that the DNP degree prepares individuals to develop knowledge generating research. It is not apparent how nursing scholarship was defined and interpreted by the participants (Udlis and Mancuso 2015). A study by Oermann et al. (2016) established that DNPs met the expectations of a faculty member, yet an area that was lacking was scholarship. Scholarship is important for advancing the nursing profession and improving patient outcomes. Scholarship refers to "nurses" active participation in activities that improve patient care, advance the nursing profession, and contribute to new knowledge (Carter et al. 2017, p. 266). Regardless of the DNP student's career trajectory, faculty should mentor this next generation of scholars in translating evidence into practice and disseminating that scholarship.

Research that is original, rigorous and significant is sorely needed—innovative 'blue skies' as well as translational research (Thompson 2009). This will require investment in the research environment as well as in people, with the attraction of postgraduate students and the establishment of a sound research strategy, structure and staffing policy. Creative, flexible career structures that link research to practice and inform education are important as well as security for capable staff (Thompson 2009, p. 696). Concern in the USA continues to be expressed in relation to the small number of students graduating annually with PhDs in nursing and the number will diminish even further if the DNP is widely adopted. Furthermore, nurses may view the DNP as a terminal degree, not just the terminal "practice degree", and will be encouraged to pursue careers in academe without gaining a PhD. Reducing the pipeline of nurses who are prepared to conduct independent research on practice and assume academic (tenure track) positions in the universities will have a negative impact on the further development of our science (Dracup et al. 2005).

According to Henly et al. (2015) it is crucial for the nursing profession to have nurse scientists from both basic and advanced practice backgrounds because they pursue different questions in their research programs. The current composition of PhD-prepared scientific workforce includes large numbers of APRNs who pursue highly clinically-relevant programs of research. This composition is unlikely if two doctoral degrees are required for preparation as a scientist, to the great disadvantage of both society and the nursing discipline (Cronenwett et al. 2011). Nursing scientists/researchers with in-depth knowledge in practice-research connections are needed to ensure nursing as a discipline maintains its voice and leadership in health care delivery policy (Henly et al. 2015). Moreover, nurse scientists are a must to ensure that nursing science is relevant, rigorous, visible and directed at improvement of health and health equity for populations globally.

Thompson and Schwartz Barcott (2019) refer to the nurse scientist as a knowledge broker who connects science and society by building networks and facilitating opportunities among knowledge producers and knowledge users. Nurse scientists are a vital lifeline for knowledge producers and users in the clinical environment. Not only are nurse scientists adept at conducting basic and applied research, but they are knowledgeable in promoting efficient and effective translation and utilisation of research so that it is meaningful and useful in various contexts to all stakeholders (Thompson and Schwartz Barcott 2019).

Nurses with a PhD are equally as relevant as nurses with a professional doctorate in the context of 'precision health', 'care between the care' and being a part of a privileged profession that participates within the most intimate moments of a person's life during their illness trajectory. Further, nurses who actively engage in scholarly work within the pillars of Boyer's domains enable the voice of the patient/recipient of the services to be heard in the complex and sometimes vulnerable landscape of healthcare.

5.6   Scholarship in Advanced Practice Nursing

Scholarship in nursing can be defined as those activities that systematically advance the teaching, research, and practice of nursing through rigorous inquiry that 1) is significant to the profession, 2) is creative, 3) can be documented, 4) can be replicated or elaborated, and 5) can be peer-reviewed through various methods. This definition is applied in the standards that describe scholarship in nursing (AACN 1999, p. 373). The Society Sigma Theta Tau (STTI) defines clinical scholarship as 'an approach that enables evidence-based nursing and the development of best practice to meet the needs of clients efficiently and effectively' (STTI 1999, p. 4). Further, Dreher (1999) hypothesised that clinical scholarship included curiosity, intellectual scrutiny, innovation, and value for care-giving. Another view presented by Schultz (2005) suggested that a clinical scholar was a risk-taker and one who challenges traditional views as inertia.

Furthermore, Riley et al. (2008) reported that one of the most distinguishing features of experienced nurses (n = 36 across four acute hospitals in the USA) sampled was their passion for nursing. This attribute seemed to drive all aspects of their work. Despite the exigencies and complexities of clinical practice, they shared in common a love for the practice and profession of nursing. Sustaining one's love for the work of nursing throughout one's career is not well described in the literature (Riley et al. 2008). This paper reported the findings of a qualitative descriptive study undertaken to describe scholarly nursing practice from the perspectives of experienced nurses in the USA. The primary driver of scholarly nursing practice, according to the literature has traditionally been the scope of work (What I Do). The participants clearly articulated role attributes as well as role processes that were integral to scholarly nursing practice. Both categories (Who I Am and What I Do) need representation in language and expectations for the development and support of scholarly nursing practice. Possessing the knowledge was insufficient—sharing it with others was seen as essential (Riley et al. 2008, p. 433). At the heart of Boyer's argument is the need to sustain a *capacious* perspective on what scholarship is, and not to narrow it down to particular forms or expressions. Scholarship encompasses 'stepping back', 'looking for connections' and 'communicating one's knowledge effectively' (Boyer 1990, p. 16).

The spectrum of clinical scholarship and the role adopted by the advanced practice nursing practitioner/aspirant is relevant also on the program of study, either Master's or DNP or PhD. Therefore, the scholarship of discovery, integration, application, teaching and engagement (see Fig. 4.1) can be seen to be enacted when the actions and outcomes of their scholarly approach are shared and made public for peer and public scrutiny. The interrelated scholarly knowing that acts across the knowledge, practice, outcomes and scholarship of the advanced practice nursing practitioner/aspirant associated collectively with reflection, investigation, collaboration, communication and evaluation needs to be captured throughout the program of study (see Chap. 6). Based on a perusal of Advanced Nursing Practice Frameworks from Canada 2000, 2008, Thoun (2011) reflected on their content and noted that the attentiveness on characteristics of practice and competencies of the nurse was unmistakably concerned with the bio-medical aspects of practice. Thoun (2011) recommended that the current dictionary definition of the word "advanced", i.e., 'far on in progress or life; complex; not elementary, and very modern' must be taken into account primarily in relation to nursing science and professional practice and not personal attributes of the nurse, nor skill sets conceptualised as nursing (p. 219).

Subsequently, Thoun (2011) posited advanced practice nursing (APN) as:

A dynamic process of *being with* others that is *guided by* the highly developed and complex terrain of nursing science, its associated ethics, models of practice, research methods, and modes of inquiry, *arising from* experience in and formal (graduate) study of the art and science of nursing, as well as the essential knowledge bases, skill sets, and competencies germane to and consonant with regulated standards of practice, and *manifesting in* professional growth, leadership, and contributions to disciplinary expansion (Thoun 2011, p. 220). Hence, in the fullness of this discursive context and thus defined, advanced practice nursing, is truly unique (Thoun 2011, p. 220).

A point of further interest made by Thoun is the notion that advanced may be positioned to describe or qualify practice rather than nursing, thus appearing as an adjective in relation to practice. In other words, and in contrast to a document title, the document is referencing advanced practice, not advanced nursing. According to Thoun (2011) although it may seem trivial, such usage has bearing on the meaning of the study and practice of nursing as a *noun* reflecting its substantive condition as a science, and distinguishes it from its most common usage as a *verb*. The attention to detail articulated by Thoun is relevant as the literature abounds with various terms, titles and confusing definitions associated with advanced practice and the noun nursing is invariably implicit rather than explicit.

Membership of a nursing academic community must entail more than expertise in research methods and techniques; it also require the cultivation of "the intellectual virtues of patients, industriousness, thoroughness and care" (Bridges 2006, p. 263). The clinical doctorate in nursing represents a significant opportunity to enhance nursing's place in healthcare settings and in society. However, the language of the clinical doctorate nursing curriculum and course content in DNP programs carries the same risks and questions raised by McNamara (2010), namely, if they are not securely grounded in nursing knowledge, will they contribute to nursing identity and the advancement of nursing or will the adoption of non-nursing language and curriculum further blur the discipline? Even if this clinical doctoral nursing preparation is built on a solid undergraduate nursing degree and identity, will nursing and thereby society benefit from the increased amount of education for advanced practice nurses? Other disciplines and society cannot be expected to protect and advance the discipline of nursing (Baumann 2010, p. 248). Furthermore, in the absence of a distinctive nursing discourse and clinical nursing expertise as the grounds of legitimacy, nurse academics appear to resort to one of the three legitimating strategies: specialisation in another disciplinary field; confused notions of interdisciplinary, transdisciplinarity or even postdisciplinarity, and genericism (McNamara 2010, p. 251).

Nursing is not merely a connection for the primacy and superiority of medicine and the inflexible construction of healthcare. Nursing, as a distinct discipline and profession, is not up for grabs and is neither arbitrary nor insignificant (Thoun 2011). Ultimately, advanced practice nursing must be conceptualised and organised within its own philosophies, theories, and methodologies. Advanced practice nurses must be prepared to foster professional and disciplinary expansion through the various patterns of scholarship that rest within and further the knowledge base of nursing (Thoun 2009). Accordingly, advanced practice nurses can then begin communicating the distinctiveness of their many contributions to the public with greater clarity and emphatic certainty (Thoun 2011, p. 220). Only then, can advanced practice nursing practitioners be courageous on behalf of patients, the public and the profession pertinent to: 'what matters most to the patient as an individual' is what matters most to the nurse. In this way, advanced practice nursing practitioners develop their professional agency.

5.7 Conclusion

Boyer integrated a broader view of scholarship that includes teaching, application, engagement as well as discovery. The preparation of advanced practice nursing practitioners informed by Boyer's dimensions of scholarship requires the development of capabilities in several areas, including but not limited to; mastering foundational knowledge; developing skills to advance knowledge in nursing, knowing how to apply knowledge to problems in practice within one's specialty and or in a transdisciplinary context and knowledge translation so that it impacts on practice.

Concern was expressed in the literature pertinent to the different entry pipelines into advanced practice nursing in the USA. That said, advanced practice nursing practitioners/aspirants will need to generate evidence of how nursing contributes to high-quality care and health care performance by developing a schema of process metrics and performance metrics that track daily activities and align these to 'what matters most to patients as individuals' and to the profession. In this instance it was postulated that the DNP can build the scholarship conduit within the realm of clinical practice. Scholarship in nursing can be defined as those activities that systematically align with the indicators of the dimensions of scholarship never losing sight of the associated characteristics identified in the spectrum of clinical scholarship model (see Fig. 4.1). The evolution of various doctorates has highlighted the challenges and also the paucity of research of their impact on patient care and the profession. That said, the dialogue on the evolution of various modes of knowledge production degrees has flagged that nurse scientists are required also, and in particular as knowledge brokers, so it seems the dialogue will continue within a spirit of scientific inquiry and from a variety of epistemological stances rather than case reports. Advanced practice nurses must be prepared to foster professional and disciplinary expansion through the various patterns of scholarship that rest within and only then will further the knowledge base of nursing (Thoun 2011).

References

Alexander S. Scholarship in clinical practice: an update on recommendations for doctor of nursing practice programs. Clin Nurse Spec. 2016;30:58–61. https://doi.org/10.1097/NUR.000000000177.

American Association of Colleges of Nursing. Position statement on defining scholarship for the discipline of nursing. 1999. Accessed from http://www.aacn.nche.edu/publications/position/defining-scholarship.

American Association of Colleges of Nursing. AACN position statement on the practice doctorate in nursing. 2004. Accessed from http://www.aacn.nche.edu/publications/position/DNPpositionstatement.pdf.

American Association of Colleges of Nursing. The essentials of doctoral education for advanced nursing practice. 2006. Accessed from http://www.aacn.nche.edu/dnp/pdf/essentials.pdf.

American Association of Colleges of Nursing. The doctor of nursing practice: current issues and clarifying recommendations report from the task force on the implementation of the DNP. 2015. Accessed from https://www.pncb.org/sites/default/files/2017.../AACN_DNP_Recommendations.pdf.

American Nurses Association. Nursing: scope and standards of practice. 2nd ed. Silver Spring, MD: American Nurses Association; 2010. Accessed from https://www.nursesbooks.org.

Austin A, McDaniels M. Impact on doctoral and professional education. In: Moser D, Todd R, Braxton J, Associates, editors. Scholarship reconsidered. San Francisco, CA: Jossey Bass; 2016. p. 31–9.

Australian Nursing and Midwifery Accreditation Council. Nurse practitioner accreditation standards 2015. Canberra, ACT: ANMAC; 2015. Accessed from https://www.anmac.org.au/accreditation.

Barkham M, Stiles W, Lamber TM, Mellor-Clark J. Building a rigorous and relevant knowledge base for the psychological therapies. In: Barkham M, Hardy G, Mellor-Clark J, editors. Developing and delivering practice-based evidence: a guide for the psychological therapies. Wiley-Blackwell: West Sussex; 2010. p. 21–61.

Baumann S. The struggle for nursing's rightful place. Nurs Sci Q. 2010;23:248.

Birnbaum R. Management fads in higher education: where they come from, what they do and why they fail. San Francisco, CA: Jossey-Bass; 2000.

Bourner T, Bowden R, Lang S. Professional doctorates in England. Stud High Educ. 2001;24: 75–93.

Boyer E. Scholarship reconsidered: priorities of the professoriate. Carnegie Foundation for the Advancement of Teaching. Princeton, NJ: Princeton University Press; 1990.

Brennan M. Education doctorates: reconstructing professional partnerships around research. Aust Univers Rev. 1995;38:20–2.

Bridges D. The disciplines and discipline of educational research. J Phil Educ. 2006;40:259–72.

Brown M, Crabtree K. The development of practice scholarship in DNP programs: a paradigm shift. J Prof Nurs. 2013;29:330–7.

Bryant-Lukosius D, Carter N, Reid K, Donald F, Martin-Misener R, Kilpatrick K, et al. The clinical effectiveness and cost-effectiveness of clinical nurse specialist-led hospital to home transitional care: a systematic review. J Eval Clin Pract. 2015;21:763–81.

Carter E, Mastro K, Vose C, Rivera R, Larson E. Clarifying the conundrum: evidence-based practice, quality improvement or research? The clinical scholarship continuum. J Nurs Adm. 2017;47:266–70.

Cashin A, Casey M, Fairbrother G, Graham I, Irvine L, McCormack B, Thoms D. Third-generation professional doctorates in nursing: the move to clarity in learning product differentiation. Int Pract Dev J. 2017;7:4. https://doi.org/10.19043/pdj.72.004.

Clearly M, Hunt G, Jackson D. Demystifying PhDs: a review of doctorate programs designed to fulfil the needs of the next generation of nursing professionals. Contemp Nurse. 2011;39:273–80.

Cronenwett L, Dracup K, Grey M, McCauley L, Meleis A, Salmon M. The doctor of nursing practice: a national workforce perspective. Nurs Outlook. 2011;59(1):9–17.

Curtis K, Fry M, Shaban R, Considine J. Translating research findings to clinical nursing practice. J Clin Nurs. 2016;26:862–72.

Danaher-Hacker E, Diegel-Vacek L, Piano M. Letter to the editor: Is it time to re-examine the pipeline for advanced nursing practice? Nurs Outlook. 2015;63:386–7.

Deatrick J. Creating a pipeline for tomorrow's nurse researchers. Res Nurs Health. 2011;34:171–5.

Department of Health (DoH). Developing a policy for graduate, specialist and advanced nursing & midwifery practice consultation paper. Dublin: Department of Health; 2017.

DesHarnais S. The outcome model of quality. In: Sollecito W, Johnson J, editors. McLaughlin and Kaluzny's improvement in health care. Burlington, MA: Jones & Bartlett; 2013. p. 155–80.

Delvin M-E, Braithwaite S, Camargo Plazas P. Canadian nurse practitioner's quest for identity: a philosophical perspective. Int J Nurs Sci. 2018;5:110–4.

Dracup K, Cronenwett L, Meleis A, Benner P. Reflections on the doctorate of nursing practice. Nurs Outlook. 2005;53:177–82.

Dreher M. Clinical scholarship: nursing practice as an intellectual endeavour. Indianapolis, IN: Sigma Theta Tau International; 1999.

Dreher HM, Montgomery K. Let's call it 'doctoral advanced practice nursing'. J Contin Nurs Educ. 2009;40:530–1.

Dreher M. Global perspectives on the professional doctorate. Int J Nurs Stud. 2011;48:403–8.

Dreher M, Clinton P, Sperhac A. Can the Institute of Medicine trump the dominant logic of Nursing? Leading change in advanced practice education. J Prof Nurs. 2014;30:104–9.

Ellis L. The professional doctorate for nurses in Australia: findings of a scoping exercise. Nurse Educ Today. 2006;26:484–93.

Ellis L. Academics' perceptions of the professional or clinical doctorate: findings of a national survey. J Clin Nurs. 2007;16:2272–9.

Fang D, Bednash G. Identifying barriers and facilitators to future nurse faculty careers for DNP students. J Prof Nurs. 2017;33:56–67.

Frick K, Cohen C, Stone P. Analysing economic outcomes in advanced practice nursing. In: Kleinpell R, editor. Outcome assessment in advanced practice nursing. New York, NY: Springer Publishing Company; 2017. p. 19–43.

Galvin K, Carr E. The emergence of professional doctorates in nursing in the UK: where are we now? NT Res. 2003;8:293–307.

Gardner G, Chang A, Duffiekd C, Doubrovsky A. Delineating the practice profile of advanced practice nursing: a cross-sectional survey using the modified Strong model of advanced practice nursing. J Adv Nurs. 2013;69:1931–42.

Gardner G, Duffield C, Doubrovsky A, Adams M. Identifying advanced practice: a national survey of a nursing workforce. Int J Nurs Stud. 2016;55:60–70.

Gawlinski A, McCloy K, Erickson V, Vandenbogaart E, Dermenchyan A. Measuring outcomes in cardiovascular advanced practice nursing. In: Kleinpell R, editor. Outcome assessment in advanced practice nursing. New York, NY: Springer Publishing Company; 2017. p. 88–141.

Gibbons M, Limoges C, Nowotny H, Schwartzman S, Scott P, Trow M. The new production of knowledge: the dynamics of science and research in contemporary societies. London: Sage; 1994.

Glassick C, Huber M, Maeroff G. Scholarship assessed: evaluation of the professoriate. San Francisco, CA: Jossey-Bass; 1997.

Graham I, Logan J, Harrison M, Straus S, Tetroe J, Caswell W, Robinson N. Lost in knowledge translation: time for a map? J Contin Educ Health Prof. 2006;26:13–24.

Gregory M. Professional scholars and scholarly professionals. New Acad. 1997;(Summer):19–22.

Hawkes D, Yerrabati S. A systematic review of research on professional doctorates. Lond Rev Educ. 2018;16:11–27.

Heasling P. Frontiers of learning: the PhD Octopus. Dordrecht: Foris; 1986.

Henly S, McCarthy D, Wyman J, Alt-White A, Stone P, McCarthy A-M, Redeker N, Dunbar-Jacob J, Titler M, Conley Y, Heitkemper M, Moore S. Emerging areas of nursing science and PhD education for the 21st century: response to commentaries. Nurs Outlook. 2015;63:439–45.

Horrocks S, Anderson E, Salisbury C. Systematic review of whether nurse practitioners working in primary care can provide equivalent care to doctors. Br Med J. 2002;324:819–23.

Kapu A, Sicoutris C, Broyhill B, D'Agostino R, Kleinpell R. Measuring outcomes in advanced practice nursing: practice-specific quality metrics. In: Kleinpell R, editor. Outcome assessment in advanced practice nursing. New York, NY: Springer Publishing Company; 2017. p. 1–18.

Ketefian S, Redman R. A critical examination of developments in nursing doctoral education in the United States. Rev Latino-Am Enfermagem. 2015;23:363–71.

Kirk Walker D, Polancich S. Doctor of nursing practice: the role of the advanced practice nurse. Semin Oncol Nurs. 2015;31:263–72.

Kleinpell R, editor. Outcome assessment in advanced practice nursing. New York, NY: Springer Publishing Company; 2017.

Koskinen L, Mikkonen I, Graham I, Norman L, Richardson J, Savage E, Schorn M. Advanced practice nursing for enduring health needs management global perspective. Nurse Educ Today. 2012;32:540–4.

Kot F, Hendel D. Emergence and growth of professional doctorates in the United States, United Kingdom, Canada, and Australia: a comparative analysis. Stud High Educ. 2012;37:345–64.

Kumar S. A systematic approach to the assessment of impact in a professional doctorate. High Educ Skills Work Based Learn. 2014;4:171–83.

Lester S. Conceptualising the practice doctorate. Stud High Educ. 2004;29:757–70.

Martin-Misener R, Harbman P, Donald F, Reid K, Kilpatrick K, Carter N, et al. Cost-effectiveness of nurse practitioners in primary and specialised ambulatory care: systematic review. BMJ Open. 2015;5:e007167. https://doi.org/10.1136/bmjopen-2014-007167.

Martsolf G, Auerbach D, Spetz J, Pearson M, Muchow A. Doctor of nursing practice 2015: an examination of nursing schools' decisions to offer a doctor of nursing practice degree. Nurs Outlook. 2015;63:219–26.

Maxwell T, Shanahan P. Towards a reconceptualization of the doctorate: issues arising from comparative data relating to the EdD degree in Australia. Stud High Educ. 1997;22:133–50.

Maxwell T. From first to second generation professional doctorates. Stud High Educ. 2003;28:279–91.

Maxwell T, Kupczyck-Romanczuk G. Producing the professional doctorate: the portfolio as a legitimate alternative to the dissertation. Innov Educ Teach Int. 2009;46:135–45.

Maxwell T. Australian professional doctorates: mapping distinctiveness: stress and prospects. Work Based Learn E J. 2011;2:24–43.

McDaniels M, Skogsberg E. The scholars we need: preparing transdisciplinary professionals by leveraging the scholarship of practice. In: Braxton J, editor. Towards a scholarship of practice. San Francisco, CA: Jossey Bass; 2017. p. 71–83.

McNamara M. Lost in transition? A discursive analysis of academic nursing in Ireland. Nurs Sci Q. 2010;23:249–56.

McVicar A, Caan W, Hillier D, Munn-Giddings C, Ramon S, Winter R. A shared experience: an interdisciplinary professional doctorate in health and social care. Innov Educ Teach Int. 2006;43:211–22.

Mundinger M, Kane R, Lenz E, Totten A, Tsai W, Cleary P, Friedewald W, Siu A, Shelanski ML. Primary care outcomes in patients treated by nurse practitioners or physicians: a randomised trial. JAMA. 2000;283:59–68.

Newhouse R, Stanik-Hutt J, White K, Johantgen M, Bass E, Zangaro G, et al. Advanced practice nurse outcomes 1990-2008: a systematic review. Nurs Econ. 2011;29:230–50.

Newman M. The professional doctorate in nursing: a position paper. Image. 1997;29:361–5.

Nowotny H, Scott P, Gibbons M. Rethinking science: mode 2 in societal context. In: Carayannis E, Campbell D, editors. Knowledge creation, diffusion, and use in innovation networks and knowledge clusters: a comparative systems approach across the United States, Europe and Asia. Westport, CT: Praeger; 2005.

Nurse P. Ensuring a successful research endeavour. The Nurse Review of UK Research Councils. Department of Business Innovations and Skills (BIS/1/624). Accessed from https://www.gov.uk/goverenment/uploads/system/uploads/attachment_data/file/478125/BIS-15-625-ensuring-a-successful-UK-research-endeavour.pdf.

Nursing Council of New Zealand (NCNZ). Competencies for the Nurse Practitioner Scope of Practice. 2017. Accessed September 12, 2018, from https://www.nursingcouncil.org.nz.

Nursing and Midwifery Board of Ireland (NMBI). Advanced practice (Nursing) standards and requirements. Dublin: The Nursing and Midwifery Board of Ireland; 2017.

O'Connor L, Casey M, Smith R, Fealy G, O'Brien D, O'Leary D, Stokes D, Namara M, Glasgow ME, Cashin A. The universal, collaborative and dynamic model of specialist and advanced nursing and midwifery practice: a way forward? J Clin Nurs. 2018;27:e882–94.

Oermann MH, Lynn MR, Agger CA. Hiring intentions of directors of nursing programs related to DNP- and PhD-prepared faculty and roles of faculty. J Prof Nurs. 2016;32(3):173–9.

O'Fallon L, Wolfe G, Brown D, Deary A, Olden K. Strategies for setting a national research agenda that is responsive to community needs. Environ Health Perspect. 2003;111:1855–60.

Paplham P, Austin-Ketch T. Doctor of nursing practice education: impact on advanced nursing practice. Semin Oncol Nurs. 2015;31:273–81.

Park C. Redefining the doctorate: discussion paper. York: The Higher Education Academy; 2007.

Parker M, Hill M. A review of advanced practice nursing in the United States, Canada, Australia and Hong Kong Special Administrative Region (SAR), China. Int J Nurs Sci. 2017;4:196–2014.

Pearson A, Borbasi S, Gott M. Doctoral education in nursing for practitioner knowledge and for academic knowledge: the University of Adelaide, Australia. Image. 1997;29:365–8.

Pearson A. The changing environment for doctoral education in Australia: implications for quality management, improvement and innovation. High Educ Res Dev. 1999;18:269–89.

Quatrara B, Dale Shaw K. Selecting advanced practice nursing outcomes measures. In: Kleinpell R, editor. Outcome assessment in advanced practice nursing. New York, NY: Springer Publishing Company; 2017. p. 45–58.

Ramcharan P, Ashmore R, Nicklin L, Drew J. Nursing scholarship in the British system. Br J Nurs. 2001;10:196–206.

Redman R, Pressler S, Furspan P, Potempa K. Nurses in the United States with a practice doctorate: implications for leading in the current context of health care. Nurs Outlook. 2015;63: 124–9.

Reed P. The practice turn in nursing epistemology. Nurs Sci Q. 2006;19:36–8.

Reed D, Titler MG, Dochterman JM, Shever LL, Kanak M, Picone DM. Measuring the dose of nursing intervention. Int J Nurs Terminol Classif. 2007;18(4):121–30.

Riley J, Beal J, Lancaster D. Scholarly nursing practice from the perspective of experienced nurses. J Adv Nurs. 2008;61:425–35.

Rolfe G, Davies R. Second generation professional doctorates in nursing. Int J Nurs Stud. 2009;46:1265–73.

Schober M, Affara F. International Council for Nurses: advanced nursing practice. Oxford: Blackwell Publishing; 2006.

Schultz A. Origins and aspirations: conceiving the clinical scholar. Excellence in nursing knowledge. 2005. Accessed from http://www.nursingknowledge.org/enk.

STTI. Sigma Theta Tau International Clinical Scholarship resource paper. 1999. Accessed December 17, 2015, from http://www.nursingsociety.org/about-stti/position-statements-and-resource-papers.

Stanik-Hutt J, Newhouse R, White K, Johantgen M, Bass E, Zangaro G, et al. The quality and effectiveness of care provided by nurse practitioners. J Nurse Pract. 2013;9:492–500.

Stew G. What is a doctorate for? In: Proceedings of the International Conference on PDs. UK Council for Graduate Education, Full Paper, vol. 1–7, pp. 22–23, 2009.

Terhaar M, Sylvia M. Scholarly work products of the doctor of nursing practice: one approach to evaluating scholarship, rigour, impact and quality. J Clin Nurs. 2015;25:163–74.

Thompson D. Is nursing viable as an academic discipline? Nurse Educ Today. 2009;29:694–7.

Thompson M, Schwartz Barcott D. The role of the nurse scientist as a knowledge broker. J Nurs Scholarsh. 2019;51:26–39.

Thoun D. Toward an appreciation of nursing scholarship: recognising our traditions, and presence. J Nurs Educ. 2009;48:552–6.

Thoun D. Speciality and advanced practice nursing: discerning the differences. Nurs Sci Q. 2011;24:216–22.

Thune T. The training of "triple-helix workers"? Doctoral students in university-industry-government collaborations. Minerva. 2010;48:463–83.

Trafford V, Leshem S. Anatomy of a doctoral viva. J Grad Educ. 2002a;3:33–41.

Trafford V, Leshem S. Starting at the end to undertake doctoral research: predictable questions as stepping stones. High Educ Rev. 2002b;33:43–61.

Udlis K, Mancuso J. Perceptions of the role of the doctor of nursing practice-prepared nurse: clarity or confusion. J Prof Nurs. 2015;31:274–83.

Volpp K, Das A. Comparative effectiveness-thinking beyond medication A versus medication B. N Engl J Med. 2009;36:331–3.

Wallgren L, Dahlgren L. Doctoral education as social practice for knowledge development: conditioning and demands by industry PhD students. Indust High Educ. 2005;19:433–43.

Walker K, Campbell S, Duff J, Cummings E. Doctoral education for nurses today: the PhD or professional doctorate? Aust J Adv Nurs. 2016;34:60–9.

Watson R, Thompson D, Amelia E. Doctorates and nurses. Contemp Nurse. 2011;38:151–9.

Wilkies L, Mannix J, Jackson D. Practicing nurses perspectives of clinical scholarship: a qualitative study. BMC Nurs. 2013;12:21. Accessed from https://bmcnurs.biomedcentral.com/articles/10.1186/1472-6955-12-21.

World Health Organisation. World Report on knowledge for better health: strengthening health systems. 2004. Accessed September 4, 2018, from http://www.who.int/rpc/meetings/publ/en/.

Career Legacy Cartography Portfolio for Advanced Practice Nursing

6

6.1 Introduction

This chapter presents the science of cartography and its relationship to career cartography. Living a career of purposefulness and intentionality can sustain long-term efforts in nursing directed at making a difference to benefit the lives of patients/recipients of the services. Career legacy cartography may also move the discipline and science forward as practitioners, educators, administrators, and researchers thoughtfully plan and achieve personal goals that benefit communities or populations. The components of career legacy cartography are discussed while being embedded in a portfolio. The career legacy mapping process for advanced practice nursing practitioners/aspirants is discussed in-depth pertinent to five dimensions of scholarship; discovery, integration, engagement, application and teaching. The practicalities of creating a portfolio step-by-step illustrated in a career legacy toolkit are provided.

6.2 The Science of Cartography

Cartography is the science of designing, drawing and producing maps (Caquard and Cartwright 2014; Crampton 2001). The science of cartography describes maps as communication devices that facilitate the examination, analysis, and conception to understand patterns and constructs. "Cartography is *Dynamic*, as it powers rapidly changing data, embraces new forms of technology, and is applied to continually changing phenomena. Cartography is *Insightful*, as maps and their users are expected to deliver insight to shape the future. Cartography is *Responsive* because map users are making and changing maps themselves, and maps are in turn causing users to change. And finally, Cartography is *Diverse* as a wide range of data, users, interfaces and problems constitute the context within which mapping is applied" (Griffin et al. 2017, p. 1). Applying the science of cartography to careers, career

© Springer Nature Switzerland AG 2019
L. O'Connor, *The Nature of Scholarship, a Career Legacy Map and Advanced Practice*, Advanced Practice in Nursing, https://doi.org/10.1007/978-3-319-91695-8_6

cartography, then, is the science of designing, drawing, communicating, and producing a map to guide researchers toward their intended career destination (Feetham and Doering 2015, p. 71).

Moreover, Robinson et al. (1995) illustrate cartography as an interactive and an interrelated methodology; "we can liken cartography to a drama played by two actors, the map maker and map user, with two stage properties, the map and the data domain" (p. 18). Therefore, space is held open for the map user to actively infer many cartographic possibilities. Instead of controlling disseminations of results, cartography welcomes viewers to undertake their own analysis, critique, and interpretations. The data/knowledge domain then transfers back and forth between the map maker and map user, with the cartography itself as a conduit. Because these interpretations depend on interaction, each viewer embodies the role of cartographer (Ulmer and Koro-Ljungberg 2015, p. 146). Accordingly, writing visually and through cartographies may open up spaces for scholars to consider research from diverse perspectives of their fellow health services researchers and from points that recognise complexity and uncertainty.

6.3   Career Cartography and the Scholarship Trajectory

Career cartography, also known as career planning, career mapping, or legacy mapping, refers to creating a visual depiction of long-term career goals and the steps or processes necessary to meet those goals (Messmer 2003). This concept is currently utilised within the disciplines of business, finance, and the wider realm of health care to guide people and their mentors chart a pathway to success. Career cartography has been described as a tool to help an individual achieve purpose and meaningful work engagement as opposed to the more routine aims of promotion or achieving a leadership position (Hinds et al. 2015).

The ability of researchers to map their scientific trajectory is foundational to career cartography (Feetham and Doering 2015, p. 72). Consequently, mapping has demonstrated usefulness for assisting many nurse researchers, scholars, and leaders define and plan programs of research and scholarship. Mapping a scientific career is an on-going, iterative, and highly creative cyclical process. Through several iterations, plans, progress, gaps, and evolving strategies are revealed. While each map portrays the key concepts and pathways for the development of programs of research and scholarship, the process is constant. Well-executed mapping provides longitudinal evidence of contributions and the deliberative process for the evidence of scientific careers (Feetham and Doering 2015, p. 73).

Mapping primarily from the perspectives of outcomes may enable nurse researchers to pictorially demonstrate the impact various aspects of their scholarship has generated over time to the benefits of recipients of health services. In addition, the process will equally be relevant for the advanced practice nursing practitioner/aspirant in the measurement of quality care process metrics and indicators. Career cartography maps depicting different aspects of a program of research can help uncover new perspectives and avenues for advancing a scientific career (Feetham and

Fig. 6.1
Conceptualisation of
career cartography
process

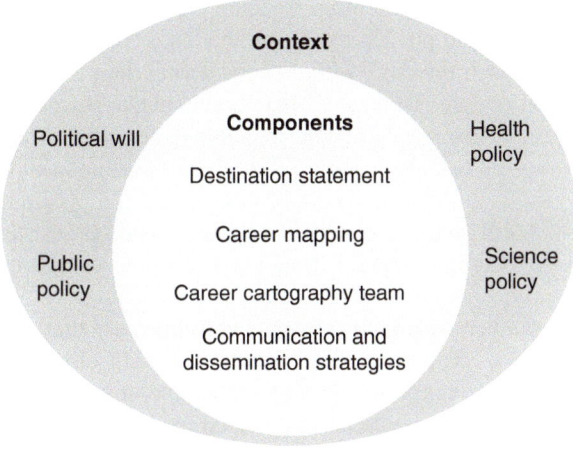

Career cartography
© Suzanne Feetham and Jennifer Doering 2014

Doering 2015). For example, a map may demonstrate the development of concepts within a program of research. Mapping of concepts helps link various activities and aspects of a researcher's program of research and scholarship into a coherent whole to make explicit connections that may not be obvious to someone unfamiliar with the scientific area (Feetham and Doering 2015, p. 73).

Career cartography consists of several components (see Fig. 6.1) that can be applied to enable advanced practice nursing practitioners/aspirants scrutinise their careers in the broadest terms, and at the same time facilitate the development of concrete plans that factor in how to move forward tactically along their career trajectory.

6.4   Applying the Science of Cartography to Advanced Practice Nursing

The goal of nursing science is to advance knowledge, improve the health of the public, and improve the effectiveness, safety, and access to health care. Similarly, the career goal of an advanced practice nursing practitioner is to improve the health of the public by generating knowledge to move toward solutions to the problems confronting nurses and their patients/clients. To meet this goal, advanced practice nursing practitioners/aspirants need to create a vision on the direction, trajectory, and expected outcomes of a career. Moreover, an active program of research and scholarship is a complex process that requires many levels of planning and strategic decision making (Feetham and Doering 2015). Furthermore, early-career nursing scientists and practitioners enter their academic positions with a multitude of responsibilities, including teaching, mentoring, research, clinical practice, and service (Brody et al. 2016). These competing demands are difficult to juggle as the faculty member is often teaching classes for the first time while trying to obtain funding and publishing. This often leads the junior faculty member to "try to make it through the day" without considering their long-term career and research goals (Holfer and Thomas 2016). Some nurse researchers/practitioners misguidedly believe that it is sufficient to be able to describe science primarily for the next grant proposal or current study. According to Feetham and Doering (2015) such a narrow view is insufficient to establish or advance a program of research and scholarship that will generate the quality, quantity, and rate of sustained change that is needed in this era, of rapidly developing science, emerging technologies, complexity of healthcare systems, and limited funding sources (p. 71).

Career cartography is a novel approach that will enable advanced practice nursing practitioners/aspirants, from all clinical and academic settings, to actively engage in a process that maximises their clinical teaching, research, engagement, practice and policy contributions that can improve patient outcomes and the health of the public. Besides, advanced practice nursing practitioners/aspirants need to develop their individual career legacy to communicate and defend their meaningful contributions to science, the policy context, and the health of the population. Achieving a desired role or a promotion is a notable career metric but may not result in the betterment of others. A career legacy, on the other hand, is fully intended to better the conditions, experiences, and outcomes of others and in the process of creating the legacy map gives primary emphasis to career contributions that are meaningful for advanced practice nursing practitioners/aspirants.

The development stages of a legacy map by the advanced practice nursing practitioner/aspirant can be anchored in a declared legacy. The first phase of the legacy map could represent the development of a program of action research aligned with their clinical speciality focus being cognisant of the policy context. The second phase could characterise the development and testing of an intervention in practice that evolved from the first stage, alongside a grant proposal submission with support from lead members of the career legacy cartography team. The next phase could incorporate transdisciplinary collaboration across clinical sites and populations utilising various research methodologies sustaining clinical relevance embedded within the career legacy cartography process. The advanced practice nursing practitioner/aspirant should appreciate that their scholarly activities will continue to evolve at various junctures of their legacy map construction, fittingly referred to by Feetham and Doering (2015), "there is neither a right nor are maps ever finished" (p. 73). Reflection on the terms "engagement" and "communities" and "patient" and "science" and "art" and "cooperative autonomy" could become a means of creative insight for the advanced practice nursing practitioner/aspirant throughout the iterative development of the declared legacy/destination statement. Then the career legacy cartography process: (i) writing a declared legacy; (ii) relating their work to current policy contexts; and (iii) situating everything together visually via a legacy map that depicts the research, professional career progress, scientific contribution, and policy context implications becomes the conduit to clinical scholarship.

6.5   Career Legacy Portfolio for Advanced Practice Nursing Practitioners/Aspirants

The career legacy map toolkit is embedded within a portfolio to capture the essence of scholarship across the dimensions of application, engagement, integration, discovery and teaching, the rational that underpins each scholarly activity, evidence of impact of such activities and a transparent trajectory of self-reflection, self-evaluation, and peer scrutiny. According to Edgerton et al. (1991), whatever its size, or purpose, if the practitioner uses it [*portfolio-emphasis* added] to build a *culture* of professionalism—professionalism in teaching, professionalism in research, and professionalism in service—you will be part of a noble understanding (p. 56). The career legacy cartography process and the declared legacy statement can become encapsulated in a portfolio so that all scholarly activities of the advanced practice nursing practitioner/aspirant can be documented and open to a process of scrutiny by peers and self, and the public. A portfolio is essentially a self-portrait of his or her approaches and accomplishments in practice; this means that the advanced practice nursing practitioner/aspirant chooses how to present him- or herself, with a series of snapshots taken over time to demonstrate his or her evolution as an advanced practice nursing practitioner. By keeping a record of scholarly activities over time, advanced practice nursing practitioners/aspirants have an opportunity to reflect on the data collected, make changes as a result, and compare the data and evidence gathered after the change has been implemented to those of the previous 6 months. Thoughtful educators and practitioners have long believed that documentation, done well, promotes better scholarship by engaging scholars more actively in making the case for their achievements (Glassick et al. 1997, p. 37). Such documentation requires rich and varied materials that the scholar and others assemble over time to make the case on the scholar's behalf (Glassick et al. 1997, p. 37). As its main goal, documentation should provide evidence that enables the scholar and his or her colleagues, even those who are not specialists in the same field, to apply a set of agree-upon standards to a body of scholarly work (Glassick et al. 1997). In the broad frame, the teaching portfolio is a container into which many different ideas can be poured. Rather than settle on any fixed view of what the 'it' is, the hope is that academic campuses will explore many images of what portfolios might be (Edgerton et al. 1991). Many universities encourage, and some even require faculty to submit a portfolio as part of their tenure application package. How to evaluate these portfolios, however, remains an unresolved issue, particularly if the task is to make a judgement about whether what is demonstrated in the portfolio reflects engagement in the scholarship of teaching (Kreber 2001, p. 285). Moreover, working through a career legacy portfolio will enable the advanced practice nursing practitioner push past the boundaries of individual local health outcomes and think about how their pillars of nursing scholarship generates knowledge that can be applied globally to the benefit of recipients of health services. Of note, Griffiths and Norman (2011) supported calls for an end to introspective research that does not build progressively on what is already known and fails to move toward solutions to the problems confronting nurses and their clients.

6.6   Professional Profile: Statement of Responsibilities

A statement of responsibilities should begin the professional profile by defining what the scholar/practitioner had hoped or agreed to accomplish. This statement establishes a basis for judging the scholar's work (Glassick et al. 1997). Using the standards proposed, documentation should address the following questions on a project-by-project basis, and ultimately, across the board:

Are the scholar's goals clear?
Has the scholar prepared adequately for the project?
Does the scholar use appropriate methods?
Does the scholar obtain significant results and communicate effectively?
Does the scholar engage in reflective critique? (Glassick et al. 1997, p. 43).

To answer these questions, Glassick et al. (1997) proposed that a "professional profile" become part of the evaluation process. This profile may have four primary parts:

Firstly, a *statement of responsibilities* for the period under review, expectations set personally by the scholar/practitioner or incorporated into a contract negotiated with the institution.
Secondly, for breadth, a biographical *sketch* would list the scholar's/practitioner's achievements in the relevant area of scholarly work.
Thirdly, the professional profile should embed the five principles that govern and underpin professional advanced practice nursing:
Principle 1: Respect for the Dignity of the Person
Principle 2: Professional Responsibility and Accountability
Principle 3: Quality of Practice
Principle 4: Trust and Confidentiality
Principle 5: Collaboration with Others (NMBI 2014)
Fourthly, for depth, selected samples of the scholar's best work would be documented to specified standards by a reflective essay and by rich and varied materials (Glassick et al. 1997, p. 43).

The scholar/advanced practice nursing practitioner should conduct a careful examination of competing activities to identify if one or more activities could be ended, handed off to another person who could benefit from assuming the activity, or done differently so that it would be less time consuming (Hinds et al. 2015, p. 213). It is essential in faculty evaluation to weigh carefully the commitments that the scholar/practitioner has made. If, for instance, a scholar has heavy teaching responsibilities, the institution cannot reasonably expect him or her to have accomplished as much in discovery, integration, or applied scholarship as those who teach fewer hours (Glassick et al. 1997, p. 43).

The statement of responsibilities might conclude with the scholar's reflections on the overall pattern of his or her work and future plans. How do the person's scholarly activities fit together, for example, and what would the scholar/practitioner like to accomplish in the next 3–5 years? How does the scholar's work help meet departmental and institutional needs? (Glassick et al. 1997, p. 43).

6.7   The Creativity (Creative) Contract

Boyer (1990) explained the essence of the creative contract; a person may devote most of his or her early career to specialised research, then the scholar/practitioner might wish to examine integrative questions-taking time to read in other fields, write interpretive essays or a textbook, or spend time with a mentor on another academic campus to discuss the implications of his or her work (Boyer 1990, p. 49). Still later, the creative contract (see Fig. 6.2) might focus on an applied project, one that would involve the scholar/practitioner in academic/clinical consultations or as an advisor to a governmental body, and a contract could, from time to time, focus on the scholarship of teaching, or engagement and or application. The practitioner/ scholar might agree to revise a course, design a new one, or prepare new teaching materials, using videos or Apps segments, for example. All such activities should, of course, be well documented and carefully assessed (Boyer 1990, p. 49).

Such a creativity/creative contract, if appropriately designed, will acknowledge the diversity of talent, as well as the changing seasons of academic life and have the capacity to keep faculty creative and productive. These characteristics are essential if education is to be enriched and if the life of each professor continually renewed (Boyer 1990, p. 42).

6.8   Professional Profile: Biographical Sketch

Evidence of scholarly accomplishment proportionate with one's responsibilities comes next in the professional profile. A biographical sketch depicts the scope and productivity of a scholar's activities and requires broad evidence of the sort that lends itself to a biographical sketch (Glassick et al. 1997, p. 44). Clearly, the biographical sketch, properly structured, can provide a detailed picture of one's professional work (Glassick et al. 1997, p. 44). Good documentation is dynamic, producing not merely a snapshot but a moving picture of the why as well as the what, the process as well as the products of scholarly work.

Within the Biographical Profile, the advanced practice nursing practitioner could engage at a higher level of capability with each of the six domains of competence (NMBI 2017) associated with quality, evidence-based safe practice and person-centered care:

Domain 1: Professional Values and Conduct Competences
Domain 2: Clinical Decision Making Competences
Domain 3: Knowledge/Cognitive Competences
Domain 4: Communication/Interpersonal Competences
Domain 5: Management/Team Competences
Domain 6: Leadership/Professional Scholarship Competences (NMBI 2017)

The engagement with each of the six domains aligned with their standards sits within a competency and capability framework of continual higher-level learning (O'Connor et al. 2018). Moreover, O'Connell et al. (2014) suggest that there is a need to embrace capability as a framework for advanced practice education. This need is described against the backdrop of viewing the complexity of the clinical environment which is nonlinear. Capability was articulated by Cairns (2000, p. 1) as "… having justified confidence in your ability to take appropriate and effective action to formulate and solve problems in both familiar and unfamiliar and changing settings".

Meanwhile, according to O'Connell et al. (2014) competency suggests a stable if somewhat static outcome because there are predesigned skills to be achieved. Adaptability to change and an emphasis on lifelong learning are thus central but are usually conspicuously absent in competency-based initiatives (Phelps et al. 2005). Of note, the term capability is reflected in the very recent definition of "advanced practice nursing" by the Nursing Midwifery Board of Ireland (NMBI):

> …a career pathway for registered nurses, committed to continuing professional development and clinical supervision, to practice at a higher level of capability as independent, autonomous, and expert practitioners (2017, p. 15).

When advanced practice nursing practitioner/aspirants engage in the "what," "how," and "why" questions posed within Boyer's dimensions of the scholarship of application, teaching, integration, discovery and engagement, they develop a self-portrait of their approaches and achievements in practice, teaching, engagement and research. Critical reflection at this stage in the portfolio can lead to emancipatory learning. Emancipatory learning is the kind of learning whereby individuals come to question the origins and validity of the presuppositions that guide their beliefs and actions (Kreber 2001; Mezirow 1991).

6.9   Components of Career Cartography

The career cartography process is composed of key components. They include a destination statement, identification of the policy context, a career map, a career cartography team, and communication and dissemination strategies (see Fig. 6.1, Feetham and Doering 2015, p. 71). The components of career cartography can be used together to generate an integrated and systematic approach for advancing a career (Wilson et al. 2017).

6.9.1   Destination Statement/Legacy

The first component of career cartography is a statement for the destination and outcome of a career (see Step 1). A destination statement is a single sentence that captures the cumulative outcome of a researcher's long-term scientific career (Feetham and Doering 2015, p. 72). The destination statement can be equated to the branding of a career so that one's contributions to science and capacity to serve a targeted population over a prolonged period of time can be highlighted (Kasprzak 2014). In other words, the destination statement/legacy is the ultimate goal of all efforts to improve health, advance science, and impact policy over time. Destination statements are not limited by the status of the researcher/practitioner, but instead are built upon a foundation that there will be full access to all the resources necessary to attend to the evolving needs of the population or outcome of interest (Feetham and Doering 2015).

Although destination statements represent the main features of one's career, they should be presented in multiple versions to reach a variety of audiences and stakeholders (Green 2009). For example, knowing how to pitch one's contribution to a policy group will be much different from presenting a job talk that highlights one's contribution to science. However, the different versions of the destination statement/legacy must maintain consistency in its message (Green 2009). Destination statements should be prepared so that they can be given in one or two persuasive sentences that give a clear vision of one's career contributions. For this reason, it is also called the "elevator speech" or the "pitch" curriculum vitae (Elsbach 2003).

Destination statements are typically refined over time and function to enable the nurse researcher/practitioner to begin mapping a strategy for reaching that destination (Feetham and Doering 2015, p. 72). Besides, Wilson et al. (2017) illustrated the starting point for their overall destination statement was provoked by asking one question continuously: "where do we want to be at the end?" Consequently, they mapped out their research projects, work goals, steps necessary to achieve the goals, and future accomplishments starting backwards from their future goals (Wilson et al. 2017, p. 345). The advanced practice nursing practitioner/aspirant may engage with the five overlapping yet interdependent dimensions of scholarship (see Fig. 6.3) and their associated indicators to navigate their thinking on the legacy/destination statement (see Figs. 6.4 and 6.5), never losing sight of the elements of career cartography and in particular the policy context (see Step 2).

6.9.2 Identification of the Policy Context

Knowing the public, health, and science policy context of a career is consistent with the science of cartography. Maps developed with the knowledge of societal power relationships (i.e. policy) results in a stronger identification of the purpose of the map (Crampton 2001). Policies are defined as "governmental or organisational guidelines about allocations of resources and principles of desired behaviour" (Trostle et al. 1999, p. 104). Knowing the policy context for a program of research is important to advance timely and relevant advancements in science and guides the destination statement (Feetham and Doering 2015; Feetham 2011).

Addressing the policy context (see Fig. 6.6) allows the practitioner/researcher position their scientific career to reveal the impact to address critical health issues in order to advance the health of the public and ascertain the best strategies for building policy capital with communities, health systems, and policy makers

(Feetham and Doering 2015). Lacking policy context knowledge and understanding, the advanced practice nursing practitioner/aspirant may follow a program of research that neither captures the political will for support nor has application or concern to the larger population. That said, if nursing science is not directly aligned with the current policy context, the researcher/practitioner career cartography will need to include strategies to inform policy makers as to how nursing science improves the health of the public and to generate the political will for nursing science (Feetham and Doering 2015). Furthermore, knowing the policy context enables the advanced practice nursing practitioner/aspirant to identify potential support, knowledge and training requirements, including barriers and enablers towards their research and declared legacy/destination (see Step 3).

Research influences change across various levels, including individuals, families, communities, regions, nations, and the global world. Thus, a conscious consideration of the relationship between research and policy is essential to demonstrate the link between research, political structures, and sustainable impacts (Villarruel and Fairman 2015). Consideration of the policy relevance forces the researcher/practitioner to be aware of all the stakeholders (i.e., patients/service-users, health providers, organisations, taxpayers, policymakers, and governmental institutions) involved or influenced by the issue at hand and to describe the impact of their science to these different stakeholders (Bensing et al. 2003).

Development of policy statements in the career cartography process can show promise for higher-level change to address a phenomenon. It can also enable access to funding opportunities given that the subject would be aligned with the priorities of the organisations of interest providing financial support to carry out the research (Wilson et al. 2017, p. 338).

6.9.3   Career Legacy Map

Certainly, as with all maps there are alternative ways to complete a journey, but the legacy map can guide nurses toward the declared legacy/destination with a journey of much meaning. Hinds et al. (2015) acknowledged that their use of the word legacy differs from its more common usage of a bequest or gift given from a predecessor. The word legacy is utilised to mean the nurses' plan to contribute knowledge, practice changes, or other aspects of health care to benefit those who receive nursing care (Hinds et al. 2015, p. 212).

A declared legacy is futuristic, and complete achievement of the legacy may not be possible, but the process of attempting the legacy will very likely be one of personal and professional meaning (Hinds et al. 2015). Together the declared legacy/destination and the identified steps to achieve the declared legacy encompass a legacy map (see Step 4 and Step 5). The map is an illustration of the declared legacy/destination statement and contains a plan that serves as a guide forward with measurable metrics and indicators to the desired improvements. In this way, legacy mapping in nursing is done with a sense of purpose and intentionality to contribute to the well-being of others through purposeful and meaningful work engagement (Hinds et al. 2015).

6.9.4 Goals

Campbell (2007) recommends when you are planning your future, you should have an overall flexible plan that will give you a range of choices, by categorising the right kind of goals; long-range, medium-range, short-range, mini-goals and micro-goals (p. 11). Furthermore, there are major factors that will influence your choices, in particular your credentials. According to Campbell (2007) with planning and effort, practitioners can mobilise their credentials (assets), improve them, and thereby expand the number of choices available in the future. More importantly, the more supportive credentials the practitioner has such as skills, intellectual intelligence, emotional intelligence, motivation, education, and broadening experiences and the more information about oneself and the world, the better decisions the practitioner will make (Campbell 2007). That said, practitioners' need to recognise their credentials (assets), expand them into the future and never lose track of the important point made; that no matter how well life goes for you at any given moment, you will never "arrive", you will only be always on the way. Live so that the "way you are on" will be your choice (Campbell 2007, p. 87).

Having clear goals also means understanding a project's scope (see Step 6). Good guiding questions help the scholar/practitioner define a project, give it structure, recognise relevant material, identify exceptions, and see new possibilities. Of course, the goals of a project may shift over time (see Table 6.2). Much of the excitement of scholarly work comes when a particular line of inquiry leads to new questions and these lead to new ones again (Glassick et al. 1997, p. 26). A scholar's goals must also be realistic, taking account of the limitations and the possibilities of the situation. Hopelessly grandiose goals may fade into irrelevancy, even clear objectives hold little value if they cannot be reasonably met (Glassick et al. 1997, p. 26).

6.9.5 Concept Mapping

The motivation and the intended end points of care improvements represent a career legacy on a format declaring what will be better in health care as a result of planned steps to create or contribute to the desired improvements (Hinds et al. 2015). Legacy planning and legacy mapping incorporate the aspects of the career goal planning literature but additionally include career meaning and purpose, which emphasise a career that both gives back to others and fulfils self. Although a legacy can be given without awareness or intent, it can be planned and made explicit with a legacy map (Hinds et al. 2015, p. 213). The literature on mapping in nursing and social sciences tends to center around concept mapping, which has been widely used for decades across disciplines (Anderson et al. 2011; Hsu and Hsieh 2005). Contemporary health care faces a broad array of challenges that place considerable burdens on the system. Therefore, processes and methods are required that can address the demanding requirements of such work and the characteristics of concept mapping are relevant for addressing problems in contemporary health care. Concept mapping has taken various forms, such as "idea mapping" or "mind mapping" to enhance creative thinking or improve the organisation of data (Trochim et al. 2011).

A chief advantage of concept mapping is its flexibility, which allows users to refine ideas and tailor the process itself (Anderson et al. 2011). Accordingly, Anderson et al. (2011) organised their strategic planning process into three over-arching stages using Trochim's (1989) six concept-mapping phases as a guide. The first stage (including Trochim's 1 and 2) project planning, consisted of the formation of a steering committee and work groups and preparation and generation of statements, or action items. The second stage (including Trochim's phases 3 and 4), generating concept maps, consisted of the structuring and representation of action items, including sorting and rating action items and constructing a series of concept maps. The third phase (including Trochim's phases 5 and 6), finalising the framework, consisted of the interpretation and use of maps. In the final phase, the steering committee examined and refined the concept maps, labelled the clusters, created two new items, and selected the top ten action items for the Public Health Road Map (Anderson et al. 2011, p. 2). Further, concept mapping is described as a standardised procedure for defining and clarifying a concept or process that is particularly useful in the early stages of describing the concept (Trochim and Kane 2005; Trochim 1989). This description supports the use of mapping for both emerging and established nurse researchers/practitioners who are planning or evaluating programs of research and scholarship (Feetham and Doering 2015).

Yue et al. (2017) conducted a systematic review (n = 13 trials) and meta-analysis (n = 11 trials) to assess the effect of concept mapping in developing critical thinking in nursing. Among the different scales used to evaluate critical thinking in this systematic analysis, California Critical Thinking Disposition Inventory (CCTDI), California Critical Thinking Skill Test (CCTST) and Critical Thinking Scale (CTS) were mostly used. The subgroup analyses suggested that concept map users had significantly higher critical thinking affective dispositions of open-mindedness, truth-seeking, analyticity, systematicity, self-confidence, inquisitiveness and maturity compared with traditional methods. Concept mapping benefited the open-mindedness, because it helped users to connect the information, accept different ideas and recognise the problem. Concept mapping affected truth-seeking through the procedure of identifying information resources, acquiring knowledge and truth. A higher score in analyticity indicated that the individual is liable to use reason and evidence to solve the problems (Yue et al. 2017, p. 93). The reason may be that in such instances concept mapping requires individuals to rearrange the existing concepts inductively and deductively by organising and correlating of the data and information, and analyticity ability could be enhanced (Kostovich et al. 2007).

The map is the visual representation of progression toward the legacy/destination statement and a clear aide-mémoire of pertinent and related projects currently in place. The depiction can also help advanced practice nursing practitioners/aspirants recognise new opportunities that are quite relevant to their legacy. An additional benefit of the visual nature of the map is that it can help guide future connections with health services researchers who have a common interest and thereby could support the efforts to achieve the legacy. Finally, the map captures and conveys the individual's past achievements and steps taken, current efforts, and future aspirations (Hinds et al. 2015). The legacy map has also been referred to as a career map in the literature. A career map is the physical document that displays the steps, processes, or components necessary to achieve one's career goals. It provides a depiction of an individual's career plan with the "measurable metrics" necessary to achieve that goal (Hinds et al. 2015, p. 212). In this sense, the career map provides the documentation that keeps the practitioner or nurse researcher on track to achieve his or her goals and can be examined on a regular basis personally and by mentors, supervisors, or peers (Wilson et al. 2017). While the career map is a very useful benchmarking tool (Tin and Wiwanitkit 2015), it requires continual attention as it is a fluid document that is frequently changing based on evolving career goals, new opportunities (i.e., funding, promotion, new collaborators), or new developments in the science. Despite its fluctuating status, the career map remains inextricably linked to the individual's legacy/destination statement, policy context, and feedback from the mentorship team (Wilson et al. 2017). Maps enable the evolution of multiple, contingent approaches to data and advance through several stages and visualisations (Crampton 2001). Maps come to life throughout the mapmaking process as well as through their use in a specific context with a specific purpose (Caquard and Cartwright 2014).

6.9.6   Placing the Legacy/Destination Statement

The first action in career mapping is to place the declared legacy/destination statement as the goal of the map. Subsequently, all outcomes resulting from the advanced practice nursing practitioner's/aspirant's past practice, research, and scholarship that inform the present research are identified and then gaps in the science are acknowledged from completed research as well as the researcher's knowledge of the state of the science and policy (Feetham and Doering 2015). These gaps become the basis for the next series of proposed studies and activities to advance toward the intended destination, which is placed both within the table and on the map (Feetham and Doering 2015). An analysis of the gaps in the science and policies that may affect reaching the legacy/destination is conducted. Furthermore, findings from this analysis inform the projected studies, activities intended and strategies necessary to address the gaps (Feetham and Doering 2015). Delineating the path that bridges the gaps from research outcomes back to the legacy/destination is the crux of the mapping process and is the most challenging and labor intensive (Feetham and Doering 2015). Developing the content to populate this part of the map may be facilitated by first creating a table to document all past practice activities, research, processes, and outcomes that inform the current research (see Table 6.1). Tables may contain, for example, a listing of methods, sample, and outcomes such as funding and publications of all completed research and scholarship (Feetham and Doering 2015). Transferring information from the table into the map is beneficial, because a visual diagram provides a clearer presentation of scientific direction and progress toward accomplishments for colleagues internal and external to the advanced practice nursing practitioner/aspirant speciality (see Figs. 6.7 and 6.8).

Mapping over time has benefits that include prioritising and organising research concepts and gaps in science. Mapping the patterns across ideas and concepts enables the advanced practice nursing practitioner/aspirant to plan the future order of studies, activities, and strategies, such as identifying needed career cartography team members, additional variables for study, clarifying concepts, and securing additional training/resources (see Figs. 6.9 and 6.10). Through this analysis, potential barriers to reaching the nurse researcher's career legacy/destination are identified and alternative strategies developed (Hsu and Hsieh 2005). The specified linkages between current and planned actions toward achieving the legacy directs the individuals' team member's attention to the importance of brainstorming (see Fig. 6.11), inclusive of the actions that will move efforts closer to the declared legacy (Hinds et al. 2015). Career cartography maps are revisited on a continuing basis as milestones toward an advanced practice nursing practitioner's/aspirant's legacy/destination are added to the legacy map (see Figs. 6.12 and 6.13). The result is a clear and cumulative representation of a scientific trajectory demonstrating progression and outcomes toward the intended destination (Feetham and Doering 2015).

6.9.7   Career Cartography: Mapping Variations

A skeleton template of a legacy map is created reflecting the components of a declared legacy, current activities, future planned steps to approximate or achieve the legacy, and a section for "other" activities (Hinds et al. 2015, p. 213). The 'other' activities contain the list of career activities that compete with efforts to positively influence the declared legacy. A careful examination of the completed list of competing activities is conducted to identify if one or more activities could be ended, handed off to another person who could benefit from assuming the activity, or done differently so that it would be less time consuming (see Table 6.3). Certainly, some of these activities may be intrinsic in the current role of responsibilities and thus cannot be ended, but there may be other ways to complete these activities not previously considered. To be a legacy map, the depiction needs to be an accurate and honest representation of (a) what is important to the individual creating the map and (b) the contributions the individual is now giving and plans to contribute in the future to the legacy (Hinds et al. 2015, p. 213).

A map can be modified as needed (i.e., changing circumstances, availability of new and relevant technologies and knowledge, and access to new opportunities) and is recommended to be updated at least bi-annually for purposes of individual career decision making and for review purposes involving career cartography team members and mentors and supervisors (see Step 7 and Step 8).

6.9.8   Establishing a Supportive Career Legacy Cartography Team

Building a career legacy cartography team is important and requires early-career professionals to know their strengths as well as areas in need of further development; have realistic expectations (there is no single perfect mentor); and take responsibility for their own career development by finding mentors and negotiating benefits, taking risks, and learning from their experiences (Wills and Kaiser 2012). Because science is a team effort, sharing career cartography maps with mentors, sponsors, and other colleagues is recommended as gaps and alternatives in the proposed studies can be identified to meet the legacy/destination (see Step 9). A career cartography team can assist in identifying the needed research team members and areas of expertise over the long term rather than simply as the next study is proposed (Feetham and Doering 2015).

Supportive relationships are critical for the successful careers of nurse researchers/practitioners and include mentors, career coaches, sponsors, and professional environments with colleagues where discourse and a spirit of inquiry are encouraged (Hewlett 2013; McBride 2011). Although mentors are often thought to be used primarily at the beginning of a career, viewing mentorship as an early and continuing phenomenon is a more adaptive strategy for twenty-first century careers (Feetham and Doering 2015). Seeing the evolution of a scientific career over time can result in defining needed experiences and facilitate the planning to achieve them. Mentoring is a way to continually pass on experience to the next generation of nurse scientists/practitioners and meet nursing faculty workforce needs (Nies and Troutman-Jordan 2012).

Creating the legacy map involves an interactive process that tends to be initially between a team leader (who is in a position to support the declared legacy in instrumental and encouraging ways) and the team member who is creating the map (Hinds et al. 2015). The mutuality of this process enhances the commitment to the declared legacy of both the team leader and advanced practice nursing practitioner/aspirant. The process of creating the map relies strongly on focused queries about current and planned future steps and listening to the response from the cartography team members to ensure that each map component is defined sufficiently and is measurable (see Fig. 6.14). Drawing the map is concurrent to the dialogue that purposefully invites reflective engagement of the career cartography team members and the advanced practice nursing practitioner/aspirant and key stakeholders.

Reflection can occur on three different levels. Mezirow (1991) distinguishes content, process, and premise reflection. An individual engaging in content reflection describes the problem and asks, "What do I know should be done in this situation?" A person engaging in process reflection asks, "How do I know that?" This second form of reflection addresses the process of problem solving. Finally, a person engaging in premise reflection asks, "Why is it important that I address this problem in the first place?" (Kreber 2001; Mezirow 1991). As a result of this cyclical process incorporating reflection, advanced practice nursing practitioners/aspirants can demonstrate responsibility for their professional development in clinical practice formatively. The portfolio would also be utilised as a summative document for evaluation purposes and the set of criteria outlined by Glassick et al. (1997) are relevant for inclusion in the context of the overlapping, yet interdependent dimensions of Boyer's scholarship; discovery, integration, teaching, application and engagement.

6.9.9   Communicating and Disseminating Science

Communicating the legacy/destination statement is just as important as creating the statement. Prominently displaying legacy/destination statements can help advanced practice nursing practitioners/aspirants outline priorities and demonstrate passion and energy for making a difference even when the challenges seem great(see Step 10 and Step 11). To advance science in today's environment where competition for resources is high, advanced practice nursing practitioners/aspirants must be able to communicate effectively the significance and outcomes of nursing science to key stakeholders. Communication and dissemination strategies that apply the principles of translating science to the public and to policy makers are as important as the other career cartography components and are informed by those components (Feetham and Doering 2015).

The research communication and dissemination strategy is a two-way process of engagement that can be responsive to stakeholder interests and result in increased demand for nursing science (Feetham and Doering 2015). Although there is no one size-fits-all structure for all situations, there are consistent elements for creating successful communication and dissemination strategies, including clear aims and objectives, identifying key stakeholders and creating memos for each stakeholder, while ascertaining their individual preferences for this process. Communication and dissemination strategies are important to advance a nurse researcher's/practitioner's ability to clearly communicate the outcomes of science to key stakeholders inside and outside of nursing, health care and academia (Feetham and Doering 2015).

6.10   Professional Profile: Selected Samples of Scholarly Work

The portfolio with representative breadth and selectivity is a way of demonstrating the scholarship of discovery, teaching, integration, engagement and application. Selectivity in the context for example, the scholarship of teaching is governed by structuring the portfolio into two major components; *work samples* which consist of the details of what was taught and what its impact was on students, and a *reflective commentary* which extends the meaning of the work samples selected by providing a context in which to comprehend their design and choice from the teacher's own point of view (Way 1997, p. 13). According to Edgerton et al. (1991) the work samples are artefacts of teaching performance, while the reflective commentary which accompanies each artefact provides the teacher's rationale for using that artefact and how it was developed. A reflective essay would introduce the projects selected, addressing their goals, preparation, methods, and results; presentation of the project; and self-critique and development, displaying the thinking behind the work (Glassick et al. 1997, p. 45).

Some scholarly activities are more readily documented than others. The scholarship of discovery, with its established system of peer review, especially falls into this category. Grants that were approved by panels of specialists, articles published in refereed journals, and books that were subject to peer review speak to the fact that the scholar's research has *already* been deemed worthy for colleagues (Glassick et al. 1997). Many scholarly activities are not so easily reviewed, such as countless hours of preparation and follow-through required for teaching and learning find their chief outlet with students in the lecture theatre. Applied scholarship often results in spoken advice to clients/patients/recipients of the services rather than a publication. Although integrative scholarship sometimes appears in books or journals addressed to colleagues, it may also be revealed in public lectures, magazine articles, radio and television interviews—not the stuff around which departmental/ schools evaluations usually revolve (Glassick et al. 1997). The selected samples needed to document the scholarship of integration and the scholarship of application is not fundamentally different from those required to document the scholarship of teaching. A reflective essay can introduce examples of best work, and the advanced practice nursing practitioner/aspirant can document the projects with appropriate materials, addressing the same standards in regard to goals, preparation, methods, results, presentation, and reflective critique (Glassick et al. 1997).

6.10.1 Challenges in the Legacy Mapping Process

One challenge to creating the map of the individual's true meaning is crafting a map that includes activities because they are believed by the individual team member to be important to the team leader. Leaders need to anticipate this possibility and speak to their sincere interest in knowing the desired legacy of each team member (Hinds et al. 2015).

Additionally, using the legacy map can be disconcerting to the team member at times because it does bring to the surface serious issues regarding professional choices and decisions and progress toward the declared legacy (Hinds et al. 2015). Ensuring an unbiased interaction during the mapping process is very important to the success of the legacy mapping for the individual team member (Hinds et al. 2015). Also, an individual team member's efforts to sustain a focus on the declared legacy can be challenging if the member's access to essential resources is dependent on one team leader who values the legacy, but the legacy is not consistent with the priorities of the greater work setting or in fact their methodologies (Hinds et al. 2015). Therefore, at the outset establishing the policy context and engaging with the career cartography legacy team and mentor(s) at varying timelines will in the long-term be an important tactic on the part of the advanced practice nursing practitioner/aspirant and conducive to the interpersonal collaborative process. Wilson et al. (2017, p. 336) described how four early-career nurse researchers applied the career cartography framework (Feetham and Doering 2015) to develop individual career maps. Despite diverse research interests and career mapping approaches, common experiences emerged from the four nurse researchers. The creation of a career map was heavily dependent on effective implementation of the career cartography process. During the experience of creating career maps, the nurse researchers recognised that the cartography process had six additional features beyond a supportive team that were critical to successfully crafting a career map in a timely manner (Wilson et al. 2017). Seven common lessons learned throughout the career cartography process included: (1) have a supportive mentorship team, (2) start early and reflect regularly, (3) be brief and to the point, (4) keep it simple and avoid jargon, (5) be open to change, (6) make time, and (7) focus on the overall career destination (Wilson et al. 2017, p. 336).

The work of Donald Schon (1983) in particular, draws attention to the degree to which effective professional practice depends not only on how tasks are approached and problems defined but also on how work proceeds. Effective professionals think about what they are doing while they are carrying out their work (Glassick et al. 1997, p. 35). Insightful reflection includes self-awareness that endures after the completion of a project. An appropriate plan of inquiry should allow for evaluation, guiding the scholar's/practitioner's thinking about what went right and what went wrong, what opportunities were taken, and which ones were missed. As part of the evaluation, a scholar should solicit opinions and show the ability to respond positively to criticism (Glassick et al. 1997, p. 35). Finally, a scholar/practitioner might follow through with activities facilitating the development of new skills or knowledge.

The declared legacy template (see Fig. 6.15) provides a visual representation of the components that an advanced practice nursing practitioner/aspirant can consider that reflect the scholarship of practice, research, teaching, engagement and integration. In order to populate the declared legacy template, evidence of a theoretical framework and a systematic or integrative review of the literature aligned with a detailed surveillance of the policy context, past and current activities could become the initial sounding platform. Then, the methods section may be the next step where dialogue with the team of stakeholders has evolved, including the planning process, and goals are identified that connect to the legacy/destination statement. The process of communication and dissemination will evolve based on dialogue with key stakeholders never losing sight of the global picture while transdisciplinary collaboration sees the advanced practice nursing practitioner pushing aside their specialty zone of comfort locally to solve problems that are highly specific in an international context. In the end, reflective critique both promises and encourages intellectual engagement (see Fig. 6.15). It leads to better scholarship. Careful evaluation and constructive criticism enrich scholarly work by permitting old projects to progressively inform new projects. It is exactly the reflection encouraged by these activities that connects separate projects and makes them integral parts of some larger intellectual quest (Glassick et al. 1997). As the advanced practice nursing practitioner/aspirant engages with the subsequent research task, the next article, the next course or consultation, older projects feed ideas to the new ones, while the new ones deepen the range of implications of those that came before (Glassick et al. 1997). This entire process is iterative, and warrants appraisal of how all the elements of the declared legacy impacts on the policy context, locally, regionally, nationally and globally. The declared legacy statement (see Fig. 6.15) provides the frame and details a sense of the architecture that the advanced practice nursing practitioner can populate within the portfolio on their career trajectory, while sustaining a work ethic of 'what matters most to the patient as an individual' is 'what matters most to the nurse' in the context of Boyer's pillars of scholarship and within a clear macroscopic view of the policy context lens.

6.11   Career Legacy Portfolio Toolkit

6.11.1 Professional Profile: Statement of Responsibilities

A *statement of responsibilities, and expectations* in each of the dimensions of schol-arship set personally by the advanced practice nursing practitioner or aspirant or scholar and integrated into a contract negotiated with the institution or organisation.

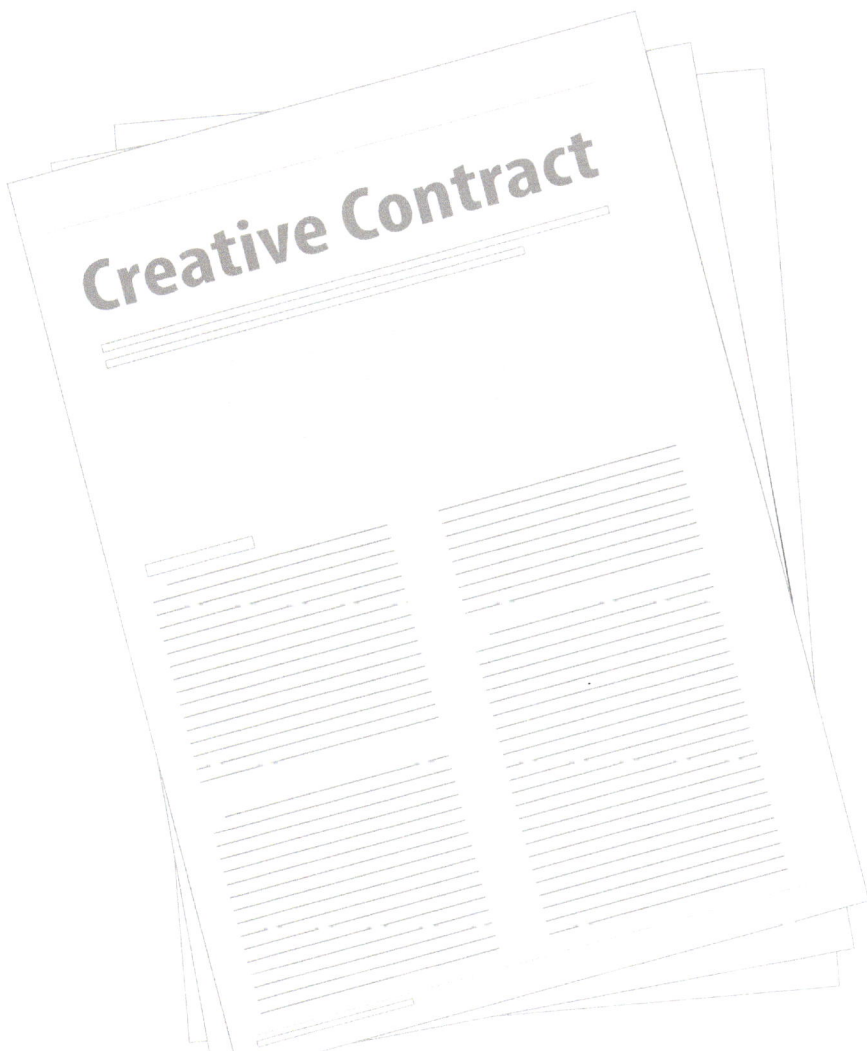

Fig. 6.2 Creative/creativity contract

6.11.2 Professional Profile: Biographical Sketch

A biographical *sketch* would incorporate the advanced practice nursing practitioner or advanced practice nursing practitioner aspirant or scholar's achievements in the relevant area of scholarly activity, i.e., practice, research, integration, teaching and engagement

_____
_____
_____
_____
_____
_____
_____
_____
_____
_____

Reflect and Complete Each of the Five Principles that Govern Advanced Practice (Nursing):

A narrative reflecting an exemplar case can be detailed with informed consent from the patient excluding any identifying details that can be traced to the case or a hypothetical case that enacts the Standards of Conduct pertinent to each of the five principles as set out in the Code of Professional Conduct and Ethics (NMBI 2014) *that align with patient safety and underpin the professional role of the advanced practice nursing practitioner/aspirant:*

Principle 1: Respect for the Dignity of the Person

_____
_____
_____
_____
_____
_____

Principle 2: Professional Responsibility and Accountability

_____
_____
_____
_____
_____
_____

Principle 3: Quality of Practice

_____
_____
_____
_____
_____
_____

Principle 4: Trust and Confidentiality

_____
_____
_____
_____
_____
_____

Principle 5: Collaboration with Others

_____
_____
_____
_____
_____
_____
_____ (NMBI 2014)

Document your credentials (assets) in chronological order pertinent to the individual overlapping, yet interdependent dimensions of scholarship

_____
_____
_____
_____
_____
_____
_____
_____
_____

Fig. 6.3 Dimensions of scholarship

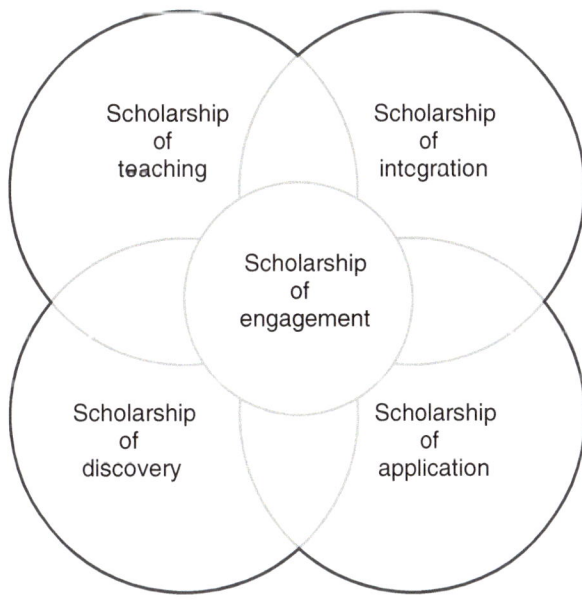

Scholarship of teaching

Scholarship of integration

Scholarship of engagement

Scholarship of discovery

Scholarship of application

Identify potential pathways for expansion in the context of your credentials (assets) pertinent to each of the dimensions of scholarship

_____
_____
_____
_____
_____
_____
_____
_____
_____

How will the philosophy influenced by your epistemology (methodology) and ontological (truth claim) understandings of the world impact on your career legacy map, scholarship and individual recipients of the health services and their health and wellbeing?

_____
_____
_____
_____
_____
_____
_____
_____
_____

Steps: Creation of Career Legacy Map
Step 1: Tentative Declared Legacy

_____
_____
_____
_____
_____
_____
_____
_____
_____

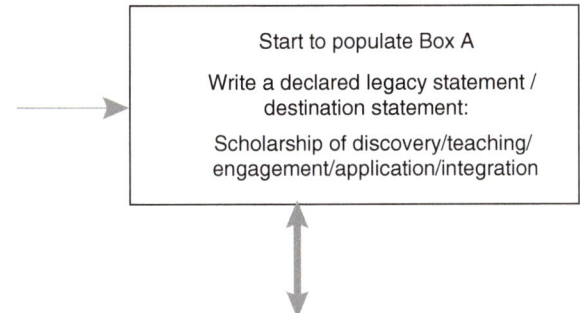

Start to populate Box A

Write a declared legacy statement /
destination statement:

Scholarship of discovery/teaching/
engagement/application/integration

Questions for consideration to populate Box A (Step 1)

1. What do you want to be better at in – nursing/midwifery /speciality area pertinent to [discovery, teaching, engagement, application, integration] because of you and your efforts?

2. What motivates you?

3. What is your passion?

4. What is your focus in order to develop the program of practice, research, teaching and engagement?

5. What would you like best to be known for by others in your discipline?

6. What lasting impact do you want to leave in your speciality area pertinent to the scholarship of [discovery, teaching, engagement, application, integration]?

7. What do you see in need of improving in your speciality area towards the achievement in the scholarship of [discovery, teaching, engagement, application, integration]?

Fig. 6.4 Populate Step 1—Box A-declared legacy

Step 2: Creation of Career Legacy Map

Develop a table (Table 6.1) to display and document all components of past activities related to practice, research, teaching, engagement and scholarship

Table 6.1 Past activities

Past activities completed	Dates	Title	Population/ problem/ purpose	Interventions/ methods	Characteristics study design/ comparator	Outcomes	Funding sources
Practice							
Research							
Teaching							
Engagement							
Scholarship							
Publications							
Other/media venue							

Analyse the gaps in the science and policy context to inform the next series of proposed activities to advance towards the intended declared legacy/destination statement

Questions for consideration to populate Step 2 [Table 6.1]

1. What have you done to date from past practice, research, teaching, engagement and scholarship that will in positive ways directly or indirectly contribute to your legacy/destination?

2. What are the outcomes resulting from your past practice, research, teaching and scholarship that could inform the declared legacy/destination statement?

3. What are the gaps from the research outcomes and the policy context that may affect reaching the intended declared legacy/destination?

Fig. 6.5 Populate Step 2—Career legacy map past activities

Step 3: Knowledge of the Policy Context to Guide the Development of the Declared Legacy/Destination Statement

Questions for consideration to populate content for Step 3

1. What are the significant public health concerns including prevalence, cost, morbidity, and mortality pertinent to your speciality area?

2. What is the political and social drive to address the health concerns of the public; short-term, intermediate-term, long-term?

3. Who are the key stakeholders that are involved or influenced by the health concern at hand; patients/service users, health providers, policy makers, taxpayers, and governmental institutions?

4. How will your planned activities; practice, research, teaching, integration and engagement inform policy to advance the health of the public?

5. How do your planned activities align with the priorities of the institution (university, health system) from a local, region, national and global population perspective?

Reflection:

6. Why is it significant that you address this problem in the first instance?

7. What are the questions that you need to reflect on pertinent to the beliefs that the problem is in fact significant?

Fig. 6.6 Populate Step 3—Career legacy map policy context

Step 4: Legacy Map Creation

Transfer information from Table 6.1 into Fig. 6.7 in order to commence a visual representation of aligning your current activities contributing to the declared legacy

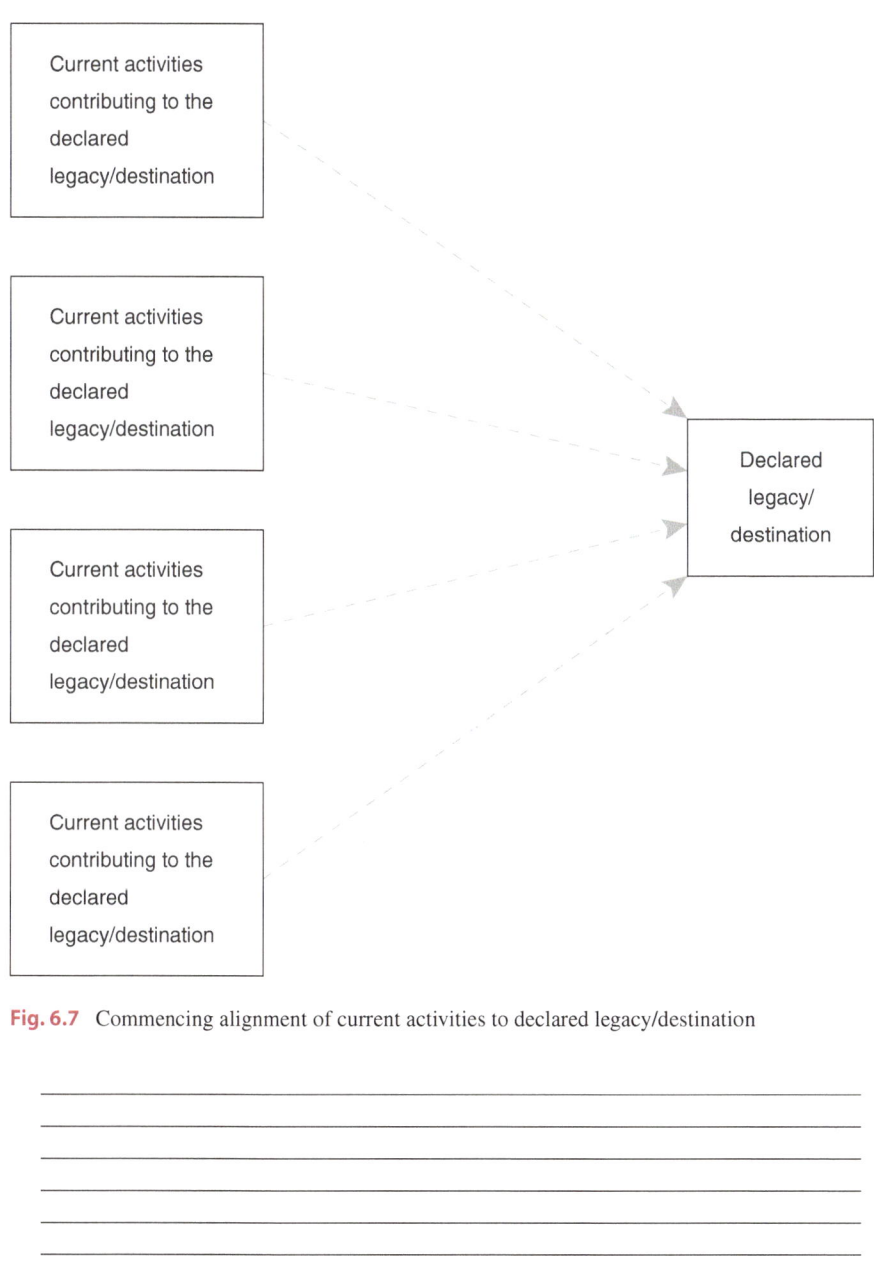

Fig. 6.7 Commencing alignment of current activities to declared legacy/destination

_____
_____
_____
_____
_____
_____
_____
_____
_____
_____

Questions for consideration to populate content for Step 4 [Fig. 6.7]

1. What material have you have already to hand?
2. What activities have you in process currently that will in positive ways directly or indirectly contribute to you being able to achieve your declared legacy/destination?
3. What are your ideas for future projects and how do they connect with your current activities and what will the end goal be?
4. What are your future aspirations in the context of scholarship?

Content reflection:

5. What do you currently do? and What have you accomplished?

Process reflection:

6. How do you know that what you do is effective?

Fig. 6.8 Populate Step 4—Current activities legacy map

Step 5: Legacy Map Planned Next Steps

Prioritise the future order of scholarly activities and strategies in order to populate your planned next steps in Fig. 6.9 towards the declared legacy/destination

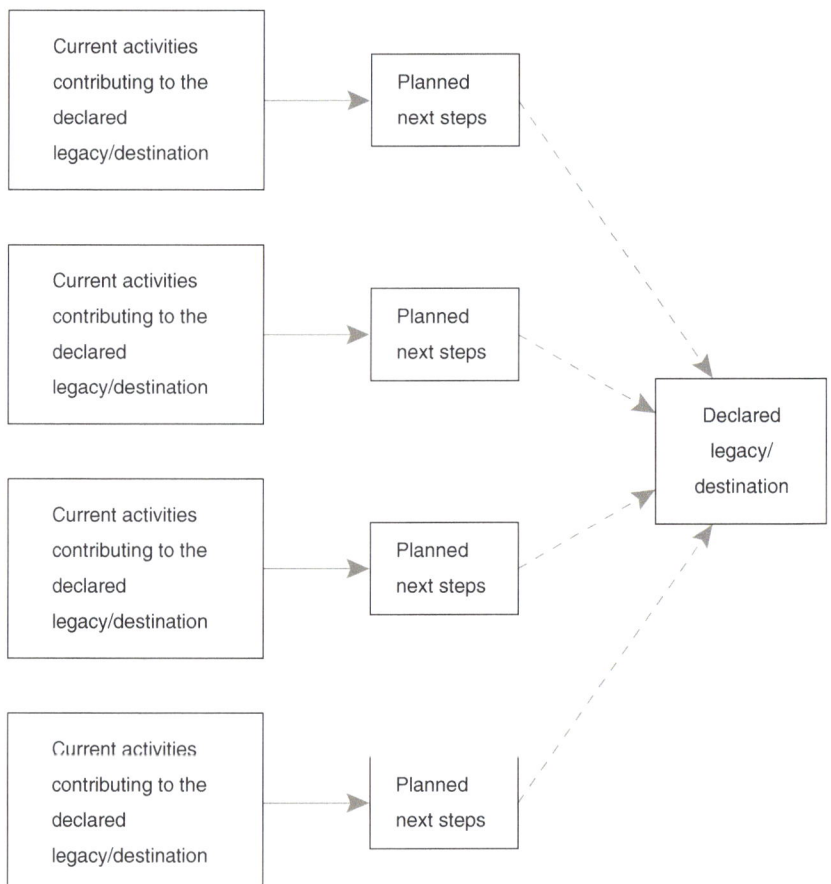

Fig. 6.9 Legacy map planned next steps

_____

_____

_____

_____

_____

_____

_____

_____

_____

_____

Questions for consideration to populate content for Step 5 [Fig. 6.9]

1. How will you get from your present state to the declared legacy/destination described?
2. Stand in the future with your legacy achieved, and reflect on how did you get from there to here?
3. What are the stepping-stones to the declared legacy/destination?
4. What are your future prioritised planned steps to achieve your intended declared legacy/destination?
5. What information have you collected for your planned steps?
6. What range of choices have you included in your planned next steps?
7. What are you willing to commit to each of the planned activities as an individual and collectively?
8. What are the links between current and planned actions toward achieving the declared legacy?
9. What training/resources do you need to bring together to move the project(s) forward?

Fig. 6.10 Populate Step 5—Legacy map planned next steps

Step 6: Goals

Identify the Specific Goals: Long-Range/Medium-Range/Short-Range/Mini-Range/Micro-Range

6a. What are your overall long-range goals?

_____

_____

_____

_____

_____

_____

_____

_____

6b. What is the purpose of your work?

_____
_____
_____
_____
_____
_____
_____
_____

6c. How do your long-range goals align with the policy context?

_____
_____
_____
_____
_____
_____
_____
_____

6d. Populate Table 6.2 so that you can fill in the gaps necessary to reach your long-range goals:

Table 6.2 Goal plan towards long-range goal achievement

Goals	Goals identification	How does that goal increase your chances of reaching the long-range goals	Timeframe	Goal status based on review and feedback
Medium-range goals (over 1-year)				
Short-range goals (1–3 months)				
Mini-range goals (Monthly)				
Micro-range goals (Daily)				

6e. What are your thoughts behind your planned actions to reach your goals?

_____
_____
_____
_____
_____
_____
_____
_____

6f. Brainstorm using Fig. 6.11 for additional pointers for reflection in order to refine your ideas and to begin to construct a series of concept maps:

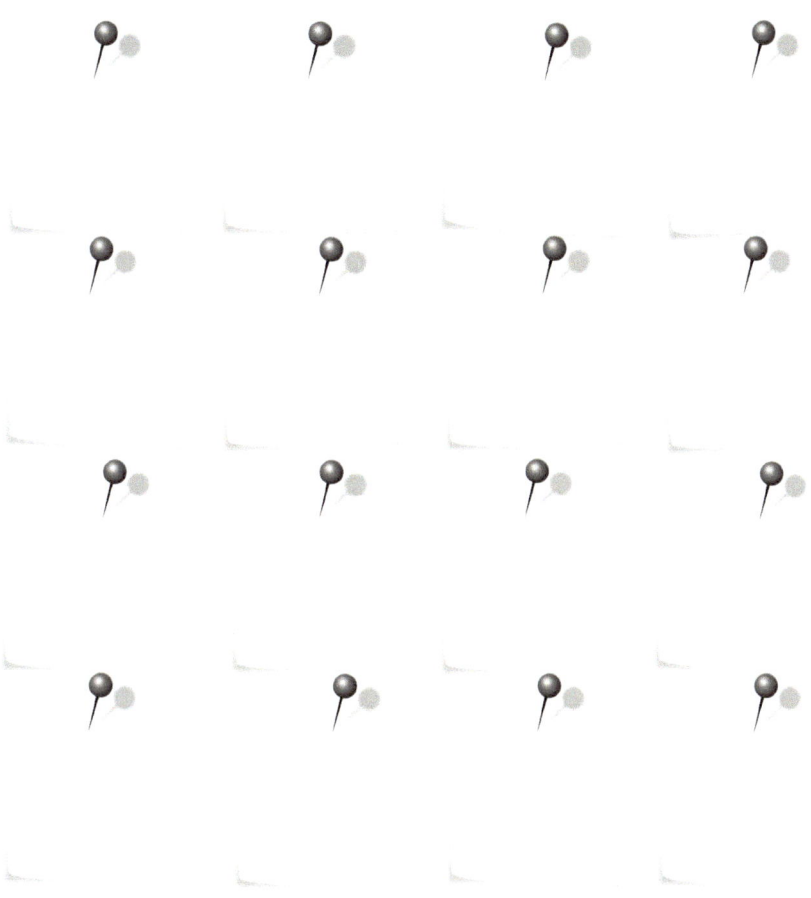

Fig. 6.11 Preparation for brainstorming and concept mapping

_____
_____
_____
_____
_____
_____
_____
_____
_____
_____

Step 7: Concept Map and Context Menu

Reflect on and demonstrate your continued progression towards the intended destination/declared legacy by populating Fig. 6.13

7a. Challenges: Action Plan

_____

_____

_____

_____

_____

_____

7b. Additional Training-Action Plan

_____

_____

_____

_____

_____

_____

7c. Planned 'Self-Scrutiny' Activities-Action Plan

_____

_____

_____

_____

_____

_____

Questions for consideration to populate content for Step 7 [Menu and Fig. 6.13]

1. Analyse, present and clarify the patterns across your ideas and concepts to plan the future sequence of studies, experiences, actions and strategies

2. Connect and group the studies, experiences, actions and strategies into building blocks and themes for your program of research, practice, teaching and engagement

3. Through this analysis, identify opportunities for support, potential challenges, and approaches to inform science and the policy context as you continuously reflect on the progress made to-date towards advancing the declared legacy/destination statement

4. What additional training do you need to achieve any or all of the planned activities and studies?

5. Create a menu to make your planned activities associated with practice, teaching, research, integration and engagement open for peer, public, and self-scrutiny

---

Fig. 6.12 Populate Step 7—Career legacy map planned next steps

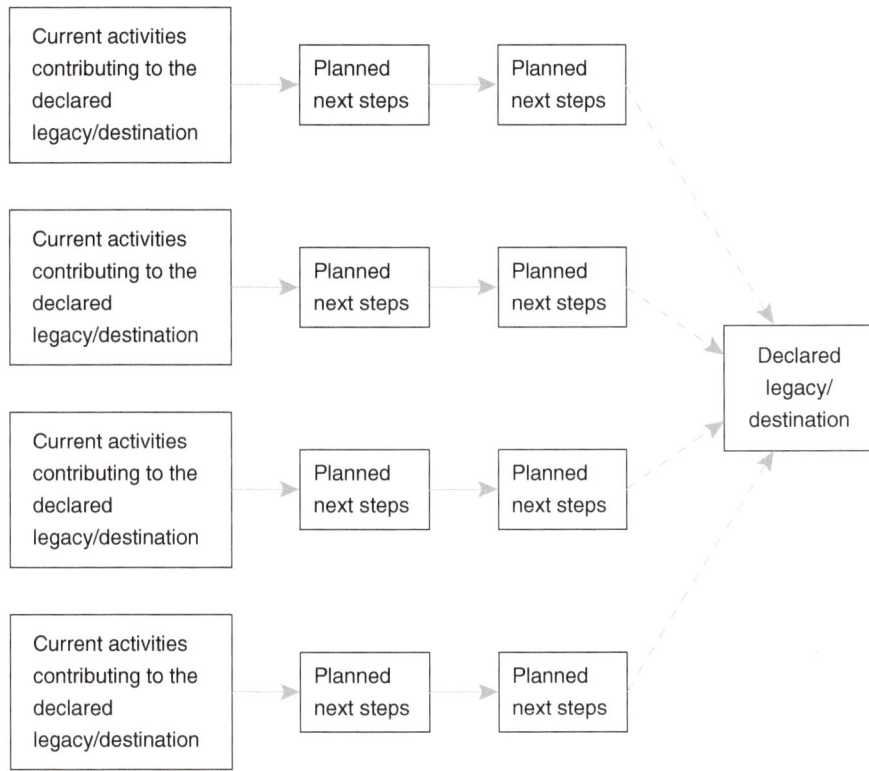

Fig. 6.13 Career legacy map planned next steps

Step 8: Legacy Map Alignment-Competing Career Activities

What are the competing career activities that do not align with the desired declared legacy/destination? Depict an accurate representation of all competing career activities in Table 6.3 in order to progress the legacy mapping process giving due consideration also of pending opportunities

_____
_____
_____
_____
_____
_____
_____
_____
_____

Table 6.3   Identification of competing activates with declared legacy

Competing career activities that dilute declared legacy efforts	Rationale for ending the activity	Delegation to another colleague who could benefit from assuming the activity	Career activities inherent in current role that require adaptations not previously considered

Step 9: Supportive Career Legacy Cartography Team

9a. Who is in a position to support you in the creation of the declared legacy in instrumental and encouraging ways?

_____
_____
_____
_____
_____
_____
_____
_____

9b. What are the team members willing to commit as individuals and collectively?

_____
_____
_____
_____
_____
_____
_____
_____

9c. What do you need each team member to do?

_____
_____
_____
_____
_____
_____
_____
_____

9d. What do you plan to share with the members of the career legacy cartography team to progress towards the declared legacy/destination statement?

_____

_____

_____

_____

_____

_____

_____

_____

9e. What are the gaps and recommended alternatives in the proposed legacy map identified by the team members pertinent to alignment of your declared legacy?

_____

_____

_____

_____

_____

_____

_____

_____

9f. What are the gaps and recommended alternatives in the proposed legacy map identified by the mentor(s)/supervisor pertinent to alignment of your declared legacy?

_____

_____

_____

_____

_____

_____

_____

_____

9g. What actions have you undertaken in response to feedback from the mentor/ supervisor of the career legacy cartography team?

_____

_____

_____

_____

_____

_____

_____

9h. What actions have you undertaken in response to feedback from the members of the career legacy cartography team?

_____

_____

_____

_____

_____

_____

_____

9i. What modifications have you commenced in response to changing circumstances; such as methods selected that require careful adjustment pertinent to the project goals?

_____

_____

_____

_____

_____

_____

_____

Step 10: Communication and Dissemination of Legacy Map

10a. Who are the key stakeholders to communicate to being cognisant of their interests and expertise?

_____
_____
_____
_____
_____
_____
_____
_____

10b. What forum do you plan to use to communicate the elements and impact to-date of the practice and science to key stakeholders internal and external to your discipline, health care services and academia?

_____
_____
_____
_____
_____
_____
_____
_____

10c. What are the significant messages for each key stakeholder pertinent to the legacy map and its contribution to your declared legacy/destination in the context of public health policy and your profession?

_____
_____
_____
_____
_____
_____
_____
_____

10d. What are the gaps and recommended alternatives in the proposed legacy map identified by the key stakeholders?

_____

_____

_____

_____

_____

_____

_____

_____

10e. What actions have you undertaken in response to feedback from the key stakeholders?

_____

_____

_____

_____

_____

_____

_____

_____

Step 11: Legacy Map Anticipated Future Steps

Reflect on what activities you might follow through-on that will enable the development of new skills and knowledge as you progress your career legacy portfolio

_____

_____

_____

_____

_____

_____

_____

_____

Questions for consideration to populate content for Step 11

What focused questions about current and planned future anticipated steps did you utilise during your presentations to key stakeholders and team members to ensure that each legacy map element was defined sufficiently and is measureable?

On reflection:

What actions did you perceive were important to undertake based on the responses and feedback from the career legacy cartography team members and key stakeholders?

Fig. 6.14 Preparatory activities for completion of Step 11

6.11.3 Professional Profile: Selected Samples of Scholarly Work

Selected samples of the scholar's best work would be documented to standards by a reflective essay and by rich and varied materials (Glassick et al. 1997, p. 43).

The selected samples needed to record the _Scholarship of Integration_, the _Scholarship of Application_, and the _Scholarship of Engagement_ will not be essentially dissimilar from those required to record the _Scholarship of Teaching_ and the _Scholarship of Discovery_.

A reflective essay can introduce samples of best work, and the advanced practice nursing practitioner/scholar practitioner/advanced practice nursing practitioner aspirant can document the projects with rich and varied materials, describing the rationale for including the scholarly projects while addressing the six standards in regard to (1) goals, (2) preparation, (3) methods, (4) results, (5) presentation, and (6) reflective critique (Glassick et al. 1997, p. 36).

Documentation should address the following six questions on a project-by-project basis, and ultimately, across the dimensions of scholarship:

Are the practitioner/scholar's goals clear?

Has the practitioner/scholar prepared adequately for the project?

Does the practitioner/scholar use appropriate methods?

Does the practitioner/scholar obtain significant results?

Does the practitioner/scholar communicate the process effectively?

Does the practitioner/scholar engage in reflective critique? (Glassick et al. 1997, p. 43).

Step 12: Declared Legacy/Destination Statement Template Completion

Populate the legacy template based on the evidence collated within steps 1–11

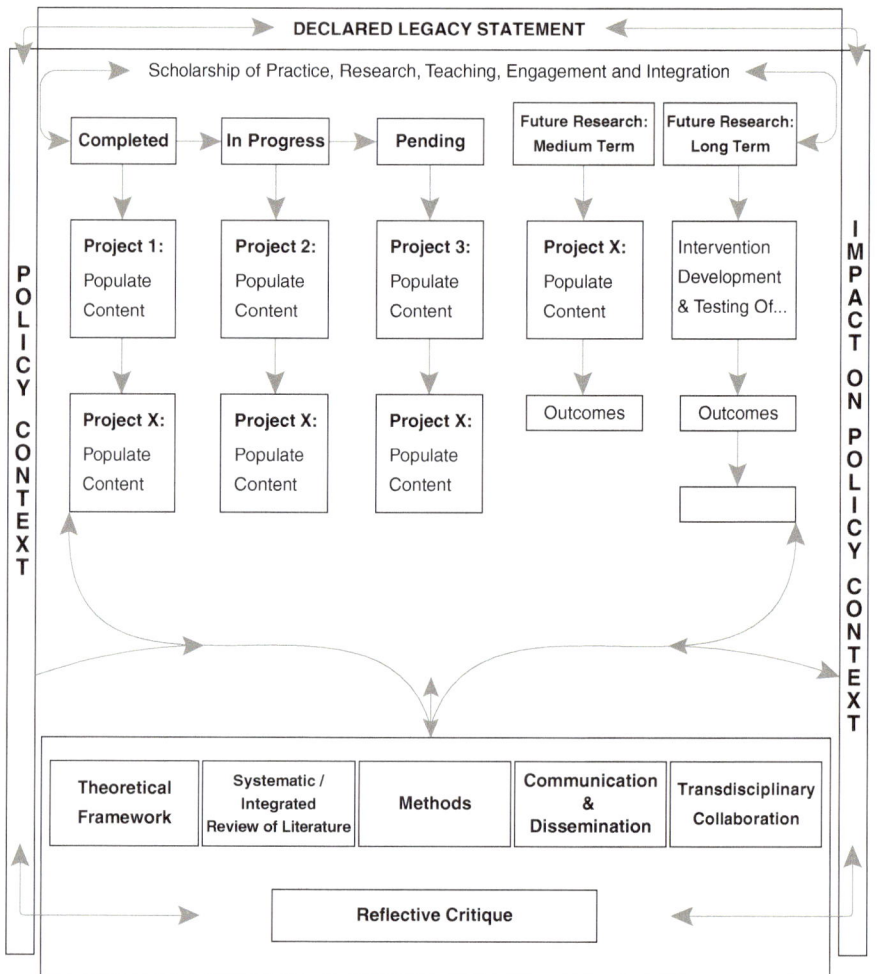

Fig. 6.15 Declared legacy statement template

6.11.4 Professional Profile: Biographical Profile Continued Capabilities and Competences

The Advanced Practice Nursing Practitioner should engage for example with each of the six domains of competence (NMBI 2017, pp. 16–19) associated with quality, evidence-based safe practice and person-centered care, align appropriately with the relevant standard and integrate a minimum of four cues with their respective performance indicators supported by current evidence:

Domain 1: Professional Values and Conduct Competences/Capabilities

_____
_____
_____
_____
_____
_____
_____
_____
_____
_____

Standard(s) Related to Domain 1 Competences/Capabilities

The Advanced Practice Nursing Practitioner will apply ethically sound solutions to complex issues related to individuals and populations

_____
_____
_____
_____
_____
_____
_____
_____
_____

Domain 2: Clinical Decision Making Competences/Capabilities

_____
_____
_____
_____
_____
_____
_____
_____
_____
_____

Standard(s) Related to Domain 2 Competences/Capabilities

The Advanced Practice Nursing Practitioner will utilise advanced knowledge, skills, and abilities to engage in senior clinical decision making

_____

_____

_____

_____

_____

_____

_____

_____

_____

Domain 3: Knowledge and Cognitive Competences/Capabilities

_____

_____

_____

_____

_____

_____

_____

_____

_____

Standard(s) Related to Domain 3 Competences/Capabilities

The Advanced Practice Nursing Practitioner will actively contribute to the professional body of knowledge related to his/her area of advanced practice

_____

_____

_____

_____

_____

_____

_____

_____

Domain 4: Communication and Interpersonal Competences/Capabilities

_____

_____

_____

_____

_____

_____

_____

_____

_____

Standard(s) Related to Domain 4 Competences/Capabilities
The Advanced Practice Nursing Practitioner will negotiate and advocate with other health professionals to ensure the beliefs, rights and wishes of the person are respected

_____
_____
_____
_____
_____
_____
_____
_____
_____

Domain 5: Management and Team Competences/Capabilities

_____
_____
_____
_____
_____
_____
_____
_____
_____

Standard(s) Related to Domain 5 Competencies/Capabilities
The Advanced Practice Nursing Practitioner will manage risk to those who access the service through collaborative risk assessments and promotion of a safe environment

_____
_____
_____
_____
_____
_____
_____
_____

Domain 6: Leadership and Professional Scholarship Competences/Capabilities

_____
_____
_____
_____
_____
_____
_____
_____
_____

Standard(s) Related to Domain 6 Competences/Capabilities

The Advanced Practice Nursing Practitioner will lead in multidisciplinary team planning for transitions across the continuum of care

_____

_____

_____

_____

_____

_____

_____

_____

_____ (NMBI 2017, pp. 16–19)

6.11.5 Advanced Practice Nursing Practitioner Schema of Metrics and Associated Indicators

Important Note: the impact of the declared legacy on the policy context can be reflected in metrics (process and outcome) and associated indicators. It may be helpful to define outcome expectations that will provide a focus to capture the relevant data

a. **Schema of Quality Care <u>Process</u> Metrics (Practice-Specific) and Associated Indicators**

_____

_____

_____

_____

_____

_____

_____

_____

b. **Schema of Quality Care <u>Outcome</u> Metrics (Impact of Advanced Practice Nursing Practitioner Care-Role Specific) and Associated Indicators**

_____

_____

_____

_____

_____

_____

_____

_____

c. **Schema of Quality Care Outcome Metrics (Impact of Advanced Practice Nursing Practitioner Role—Health Care Organisation Target Specific) and Associated Indicators**

_____
_____
_____
_____
_____
_____
_____
_____
_____

Additional component to complete the portfolio: Reflection on how the quality care process and outcome metrics and associated indicators may be translated into sustained improvement that meets the healthcare needs of the population as a direct result of the advanced practice nursing practitioner's scholarly practice

_____
_____
_____
_____
_____
_____
_____
_____
_____

6.12 Conclusion

Career cartography, also known as career planning, career mapping, or legacy mapping, refers to creating a visual depiction of long-term career goals and steps or processes necessary to meet those goals (Messmer 2003). Career cartography consists of several components that can be applied to enable advanced practice nursing practitioner/aspirants scrutinise their careers in the broadest terms, and at the same time facilitate the development of concrete plans that factor in how to move forward tactically along the trajectory of each of the dimensions of scholarship, namely, discovery, teaching, integration, application and engagement. Career cartography is presented in detail embedded in a portfolio as a novel approach that will enable advanced practice nursing practitioners/aspirants from all clinical/academic settings, to actively engage in a process that maximises their clinical teaching, research, engagement, practice and policy context contributions that can improve outcomes for the recipients of the services and promote the health of the population. Seven lessons reported in the literature pertinent to the creation of the career legacy cartography process are outlined which serve as a reminder to the challenges associated in the design and implementation of the legacy/destination statement. A template is presented exemplifying a legacy statement diagram that will provide cues to the advanced practice nursing practitioner/aspirant on the elements involved in such a representation. Further, transparency in the scientific evidence brokered by the advanced practice nursing practitioner as it relates to the policy context and outcomes becomes a building block for transdisciplinary collaboration without losing sight of the clinical context where the patient/recipient of the service is placed front and centre within the spectrum of clinical scholarship, governance and accountability.

References/Bibliography

Appendices of Portfolio

- **Contract**
- **Business Case and Implementation Plan**
- **Job Description Aligned to Standards and Domains of Professional**
- **Business Case and Implementation Plan**

Advanced Nursing Practice

- **Scope of Professional and Expert Practice Decision Analysis Algorithms**
- **PRISMA Template of Database Sources Searched for Individual Research Projects**

References

Anderson L, Day K, Vandenberg A. Using a concept map as a tool for strategic planning. The healthy brain initiative. Prev Chronic Dis. 2011;8:A117. PMC3181190.

Bensing J, Caris-Verhallen W, Dekker J, Delnoij D, Groenewegen P. Doing the right thing and doing it right: toward a framework for assessing the policy relevance of health services research. Int J Technol Assess Health Care. 2003;19:604–12.

Boyer E. Scholarship reconsidered: priorities of the professoriate. Carnegie Foundation for the Advancement of Teaching. Princeton, NJ: Princeton University Press; 1990.

Brody A, Edelman L, Siegel E, Foster V, Bailey D, Leak Bryant A, Bond S. Evaluation of a peer mentoring program for early career gerontological nursing faculty and its potential for application to other fields in nursing and health sciences. Nurs Outlook. 2016;64:332–8.

Cairns L. The process/outcome approach to becoming a capable organisation. Australian Capability Network Conference, Sydney Australia; 2000. p. 1–14.

Campbell DP. If you don't know where you're going you'll end up somewhere else. Notre Dame, IN: Sorin Books; 2007.

Caquard S, Cartwright W. Narrative cartography: from mapping stories to the narrative of maps and mapping. Cartogr J. 2014;51:101–6.

Crampton J. Maps as social construction: power, communication and visualisation. Progr Hum Geogr. 2001;25:235–52.

Edgerton R, Hutchings P, Quinlan K. The Teaching portfolio: capturing the scholarship of teaching. Washington, DC: American Association for Higher Education; 1991.

Elsbach K. How to pitch a brilliant idea. Harv Bus Rev. 2003;81:117–23.

Feetham S. The role of science policy in programs of research and scholarship. In: Hinshaw AS, Grady PA, editors. Shaping health policy through nursing research. New York, NY: Springer; 2011. p. 53–72.

Feetham S, Doering J. Career cartography: a conceptualisation of career development to advance health policy. J Nurs Scholarsh. 2015;47:70–7.

Glassick C, Huber M, Maeroff G. Scholarship assessed: evaluation of the professoriate. San Francisco, CA: Jossey-Bass; 1997.

Green H. Destination statement: getting from here to where you want to go. 2009. Accessed from http://thehumanfactor.biz/wordpress/wp-content/uploads/2009/07/1209-smart-people-destina-tion-statement.pdf.

Griffin A, Robinson A, Roth R. Envisioning the future of cartographic research. Int J Cartogr. 2017;3:1–8.

Griffiths P, Norman I. What is a nursing research journal? Int J Nurs Stud. 2011;47:1311–4.

Hewlett S. Forget a mentor, find a sponsor: the new way to fast track your career. Boston, MA: Harvard Business School Publishing; 2013.

Hinds P, Britton D, Coleman L, Engh E, Humbel T, Keller S, Walczak D. Creating a career legacy map to help assure meaningful work in nursing. Nurs Outlook. 2015;63:211–8.

Holfer L, Thomas K. Transition of new graduate nurses to the workforce: challenges and solutions in the changing health care environment. N C Med J. 2016;77:133–6.

Hsu L, Hsieh S. Concept maps as an assessment tool in a nursing course. J Prof Nurs. 2005;21: 141–9.

Kasprzak L. Build your brand for positive career impact. Chem Eng Prog. 2014;110:25.

Kostovich C, Poradzisz M, Wood K, O'Brien K. Learning style preference and student aptitude for concept maps. J Nurs Educ. 2007;46:225–31.

Kreber C. Designing teaching portfolios based on a formal model of the scholarship of teaching. To improve the academy. J Educ Dev. 2001;19:285–305.

McBride A. The growth and development of nurse leaders. New York, NY: Springer; 2011.

Messmer M. Career mapping: charting an employee's path to success. Strat Finan. 2003;83:1–2.

Mezirow J. Transformative dimensions of adult learning. San Francisco, CA: Jossey-Bass; 1991.

Nies M, Troutman-Jordan M. Mentoring nurse scientists to meet nursing faculty workforce needs. Scientific World Journal. 2012;2012:345085. https://doi.org/10.1100/2012/345085. 5 pages.

Nursing and Midwifery Board of Ireland (NMBI). Code of professional conduct and ethics for registered nurses and registered midwives. Dublin: The Nursing and Midwifery Board of Ireland; 2014.

Nursing and Midwifery Board of Ireland (NMBI). Advanced practice (nursing) standards and requirements. Dublin: The Nursing and Midwifery Board of Ireland; 2017.

O'Connell J, Gardner G, Coyer F. Beyond competencies: using a capability framework in developing practice standards for advanced practice nursing. J Adv Nurs. 2014;70:2728–35.

O'Connor L, Casey M, Smith R, Fealy G, O'Brien D, O'Leary D, Stokes D, McNamara M, Glasgow ME, Cashin A. The universal, collaborative and dynamic model of specialist and advanced nursing and midwifery practice: a way forward? J Clin Nurs. 2018;27:e882–94.

Phelps R, Haas S, Ellis A. Competency, capability, complexity and computers: exploring a new model for conceptualising end-user computer education. Br J Educ Technol. 2005;36:67–84.

Robinson A, Morrison J, Muehrcke P, Kimerling A, Guptill S. Elements of cartography. New York, NY: John Wiley; 1995.

Schon D. The reflective practitioner. New York, NY: Basic Books Inc., Publishers; 1983.

Tin S, Wiwanitkit V. Career legacy map. Nurs Outlook. 2015;63:109.

Trochim W. Concept mapping: soft science or hard art? Eval Program Plann. 1989;12:87–110.

Trochim W, Kane M. Concept mapping: an introduction to structured conceptualisation in health care. International J Qual Health Care. 2005;17:187–91.

Trochim W, Kane C, Graham M, Pincus H. Evaluating translational research: a process marker model. Clin Transl Sci. 2011;4:153–62.

Trostle J, Bronfaman M, Langer A. How do researchable influence decision-makers? Case studies of Mexican policies. Health Policy Plan. 1999;14:103–14.

Ulmer J, Koro-Ljungberg M. Writing visually through (methodological) events and cartography. Qual Inq. 2015;2:138–52.

Villarruel A, Fairman J. The Council for the Advancement of Nursing Science, Idea Festival advisory committee: good ideas that need to go further. Nurs Outlook. 2015;63:436–8.

Way D. Teaching evaluation handbook. Ithaca, NY: Cornell University Center for Teaching Excellence, Cornell University; 1997.

Wills C, Kaiser L. Navigating the course of scholarly productivity: the protégé role in mentoring. Nurs Outlook. 2012;50:61–6.

Wilson D, Rosemberg M, Visovatti M, Munro-Kramer M, Feetham S. Career cartography: from stories to science and scholarship. J Nurs Scholarsh. 2017;49:336–46.

Yue M, Zhang M, Zhang C, Jin C. The effectiveness of concept mapping on development of critical thinking in nursing education: a systematic review and meta-analysis. Nurse Educ Today. 2017;52:87–94.

Reflections of a 'Joint Clinical Chair-Advanced Practice Nursing Practitioner' on Finding Meaning in a Patient's Story Allied with Clinical Scholarship

7

7.1 Introduction

An exemplar case in clinical practice is explored by a joint-chair of clinical nursing (clinical professor). The complexity of the pain case is unraveled utilising a patient-centered framework. The meaning of the patient story is narrated through the lens of the clinical professor who is also an advanced practice nursing practitioner with prescriptive authority in pain medicine. The capabilities expected of a clinical professor in practice are put to the test as the case unfolds. The outcome hopefully will provoke conversation among advanced practice nursing practitioners/aspirants on the enablers that nurses bring to the bedside in the context of 'what matter most to the patient as an individual' is 'what matters most to the nurse'. Nurses are clinically committed to help their patients, and this help entails curative efforts to alleviate patient suffering, as well as looking after their well-being in a concerned attitude of care that is quintessential to the clinical encounter (Kottow 2001, p. 60).

7.1.1 Exemplar Case and Context

The case is based on Jamie, a 53 year old male with a 5 year history of severe pain over the cervical spine and right shoulder in the T1 distribution. Jamie has a long-standing history of low back pain. He also had in the past [3 years prior] a herpetic lesion on the lip associated with pain mainly in the occipital region consistent with the occipital nerve which originates mostly from C2 bilaterally. There were areas of scarring with hyperalgesia and allodynia consistent with post-herpetic neuralgia. The provisional diagnosis is Cervical Spondylosis. He is attending a scheduled appointment at a large academic medical centre for a high-tech pain infusion. The main complaint is interscapular pain, radiating to right neck and skull base, atypical chest pain, tiredness and exhaustion, of 3–5 years duration.

© Springer Nature Switzerland AG 2019

L. O'Connor, *The Nature of Scholarship, a Career Legacy Map and Advanced Practice*, Advanced Practice in Nursing, https://doi.org/10.1007/978-3-319-91695-8_7

The significant past history revealed a fall 12 years ago, head injury, right shoulder and neck injury, and fractured ribs. Neck surgery was for significant neck pain, interscapular pain and tingling and numbness in the middle fingers of the right hand, for which Jamie underwent spinal surgery at C6/7 level 7 years ago. The symptoms in the right arm were relieved following the surgery, but this was followed by an exacerbation of interscapular pain. The longstanding low back pain remains central, usually one episode a week, no specific trigger, no radicular symptoms and no radiculopathy. Over the months Jamie also gave a history of sharp pain in the right ear and also pain in the occipital region. Over the last 3 years Jamie has had repeated admissions to hospital with atypical chest pain, thoroughly investigated, not of cardiac origin, last review for this atypical pain was 2 weeks prior to this clinical encounter. He has several risk factors including a high cholesterol, family history of ischaemic heart disease and a cigarette smoker.

On direct questioning by the advanced practice nursing practitioner prior to commencing the high-tech pain infusion, it seems that the pain extending all the way down the right arm is ongoing but the intermittent numbness has substantially improved since the cervical spine surgery 7 years ago. The symptoms appear to be present at all times, but deteriorate considerably by the middle of the day and by the end of the day Jamie reports feeling exhausted. In addition, Jamie reports both arms and legs become weak, and sometimes he thinks he does not have the strength to drive the short distance home. He tends to lie down and rest a lot and has had repeated pain interventions [nerve blocks] over the course of the last 3 years with minimal effect and no improvement in quality of life. On examination, Jamie was generally fit and healthy, a smoker of 20–25 nicotine cigarettes a day, and has a high cholesterol. He had normal tone and power in both upper limbs. He is an independent and ambulatory gentleman. He, however did have an area of tenderness in the interscapular regions, slightly on the right side of the mid-line, directly opposite the T1–T3 spinous processes. A very restricted neck movement was noted on formal assessment, at other times neck movements seemed quite good spontaneously. Well healed neck wound was identified pertinent to the cervical surgery. No motor or sensory loss. No reduction of supinator reflexes. A post-operative MRI scan [7 years ago] showed satisfactory decompression at the operated level, and subsequent MRI [6 months ago] revealed no other evidence of spinal cord or root compression in the adjacent levels. An MRI Brain was within normal limits and a neurology opinion was sought 1 year ago, but nothing focal could be detected. Overall the current symptoms are difficult to explain and correlate with his associated signs. The symptoms seem to be musculoskeletal in origin and are not explainable by a normal dermatomal pattern of ongoing symptoms.

Chronic pain has been recognized as pain that persists past normal healing time (Bonica 1953) and therefore lacks the acute warning function of physiological nociception. Usually pain is regarded as chronic when it lasts or recurs for more than 3 months (Treede et al. 2015; Merskey and Bogduk 1994). Chronic pain should receive greater attention as a global health priority because adequate pain treatment is a human right, and it is the duty of any health care system to provide it (Goldberg and Summer 2011; Bond et al. 2006). Furthermore, chronic pain is a frequent condition, affecting an estimated 20% of the population worldwide (Van Hecke et al. 2013; Goldberg and Summer 2011; IOM 2011; Schopflocker et al. 2011; Gureje et al. 2008; Breivik et al. 2006). Besides, a classification for chronic primary pain has been introduced and defined as pain in one or more anatomical regions that

(1) Persists or recurs for longer than 3 months
(2) Is associated with significant emotional distress (e.g., anxiety, anger, frustration, or depressed mood) and/or significant functional disability (interference in activities of daily life and participation in social roles) and
(3) The symptoms are not better accounted for by another diagnosis (Nicholas et al. 2019, p. 29).

Comorbidity between chronic pain and other conditions, such as psychiatric conditions, has been well documented (Kirsh 2010). The presence of comorbid conditions is important, as there is evidence that health-care utilisation and health-care costs increase and health-related quality of life diminishes (Dominick et al. 2012). Specific to pain comorbidities, patients with multiple pain sites or pain syndromes also report higher levels of anxiety and depressive symptoms (Gore et al. 2012; Gureje et al. 2008). A recent study found that a third of patients reported coexisting chronic pain conditions, but no specific patterns of co-occurrence of pain comorbidity were identified (Page et al. 2018). Furthermore, the presence of coexisting pain conditions was found to be significantly associated with lower quality of life, longer pain duration, and older age. In addition, the presence of co-existing chronic pain diagnoses did not seem to have a clinically significant impact on treatment responses (Page et al. 2018).

7.1.2 Exemplar Case and the Role of the Advanced Practice Nursing Practitioner

A Joint Clinical Chair usually refers to a professorial position which is a joint appointment between a university, school, college or faculty and a health service organisation, although there are many different models. In this case, the Joint Clinical Chair involved two major academic medical centres and one large university. According to Darbyshire (2010) establishing a joint chair position is a significant, important organisational initiative and investment on the part of the university and hospital. The process should be trusted and the professor left alone to undertake the day-to-day activities. If the selection process has been rigorous and carefully considered, then the successful applicant will be more than capable of being a self-starter, using their creativity, showing imagination rather than always demanding resources, developing the role and their department in exciting and valuable ways, and meeting the aims and goals of the position (Darbyshire 2010). This is why the appointment is at professorial level. This is what the person has been hired to do, not to undertake the minutiae of another's agenda (Darbyshire 2010, p. 2598).

In this exemplar case, the role of Joint Clinical Chair enabled each of the five dimensions of scholarship as outlined by Boyer namely, scholarship of teaching, discovery, integration, application and engagement weave through her role as a registered advanced nursing practitioner with prescriptive authority in pain medicine. The flexible bridges between clinical and academia merged and were filled with opportunities. The visibility of the registered advanced practice nursing practitioner (RANP) with prescriptive authority (RNP) at the bedside doing and thinking pain management with a title 'clinical professor, RANP, RNP, PhD' was a game-changer for the clinical staff, the clinical professor and more importantly the patient. The elements of a professional triad of 'expertise, clinical scholarship and scholarly activity' were viewed as a valuable resource in the clinical setting. Moreover, the infiltration of this professional triad without pomp or ceremony, respecting the clinical knowledge base at the bedside and that of the patient rightly connected the elements of the triad and engineered and implemented a program of research grounded in actual practice.

7.2   Reflection Through the Lens of a 'Joint Clinical-Chair-Advanced Practice Nursing Practitioner'

This exemplar case will be framed in a person-centered framework adapting Mead and Bower's (2000) work and weaving each of their dimensions throughout the case. According to the aforementioned authors, a patient-centered approach is increasingly regarded as crucial for the delivery of high quality care by doctors; the adaptation to nurses in this exemplar case will be presented. The adaptations of the five dimensions are as follows: 'biopsychosocial perspective', 'the patient-as-person', 'sharing power and responsibility', 'the therapeutic alliance', and 'the nurse-as-person' (Mead and Bower 2000).

Jamie presented for a high-tech infusion for severe right neck pain, right shoulder pain and right arm pain. This was the ninth infusion that occurred weekly. He reported varying response to the preceding infusions which were captured in a pain diary that was part of the weekly pain management evaluation plan. Infusion 8 provided 2 days moderate pain relief [right neck, right arm, and right shoulder], approximately 30% reduction of pain that afforded two nights of restful sleep, reduction in fatigue and moderate improvement in functional status. Of note, the atypical central chest pain was reported to be always present, a continuous feature over the course of the last 3 years that was investigated extensively by various cardiology teams.

A thorough and detailed current pain history was completed to ascertain the characteristics of the pain; associated symptoms, precipitating factors and palliation, quality, region, radiation, risk factors, red flags, sensation, severity, source, epicentre, patient expectations, relationship with others, enjoyment of life, mood, sleep, support system at home, walking, activities, working life, and any evidence of trauma. In addition, current pain symptoms over the last 24 h and over the previous 2 weeks were explored with Jamie, plus any subtle changes in the pattern, any new pain/

stiffness/aching/hurting/soreness or discomfort. Because chronic pain is a complex phenomenon resulting from many factors including biological, psychological and social factors (Pizzo and Clarke 2012), all aspects were incorporated in the pain history. Understanding the patients' illnesses in general within a broader 'biopsychosocial perspective' is one of the dimensions of patient-centered care (Mead and Bower 2000). The biopsychosocial model provides an ideal framework for conceptualising individual differences in pain. This model posits that the experience of pain is influenced by complex and dynamic interactions among multiple biological, psychological, and social factors (Gatchel et al. 2007). Importantly, the ensemble of biopsychosocial factors contributing to the experience of pain and its expression varies considerably across people. Thus pain is sculpted by a mosaic of factors that is completely unique to each individual at a given point in time, and this mosaic must be considered to provide optimal pain treatment (Fillingham 2017, p. S11).

In the narratives that construct patient-centeredness as a process of caring, healthcare professionals are required to adopt the biopsychosocial model, which Tanenbaum (2013) encapsulates as caring for the whole person instead of their parts. The healthcare professional needs to see patients as persons who experience their illness individually, within their unique social setting (Illingworth 2010). Hence health care professionals are urged to take a holistic perspective and to pay attention to the patient's illness experience:

> Holistic care recognises and values whole persons as well as the interdependence of their parts. The whole person is described as the biological, social, psychological, and spiritual aspects of a person. Providing holistic care allows the clinician to better understand how an illness affects the entire person (Mead and Bower 2000).

From a holistic perspective, what was it that advanced practice nursing practitioner noticed? A change in the pattern of pain, even though Jamie emphasised that there was no change, no difference, no new symptoms, the same reduction in reported quality of life due to pain and the affect of that pain. In fact, Jamie queried why the advanced practice nursing practitioner continued to question him about the pain when the answers he would give would be identical. He repeatedly emphasised being weary of reiterating the details even though the advanced practice nursing practitioner approached the assessment like rehearsing and reassembling the chunks in a holistic way to unpack the sense that there was something different in the detail, but it was nothing specific, and physiological cues were all within normal parameters. It felt like on-the-spot experimenting, referred to as reflection-in-action (Schon 1983), generating an informal theory and testing a hypothesis in this practice situation. Every detail was attended to in a systematic way; ascertain his expectations, preferences, needs, and his interpretation of the pain, hopes and feelings and relating each element of the findings to Jamie. I was acutely aware that Jamie clearly expressed that he was in the department of pain medicine for the high tech pain infusion today and that plan was not open for renegotiation as the pain characteristics were unchanged from the previous weeks. Jamie also indicated that the high tech pain infusion gave him hope, even though it was short-lived but relevant to him. The second dimension of person-centered care is concerned with 'understanding the individual's experience of illness' (Mead and Bower 2000). The key here is trying to understand Jamie's self-report of pain and the symptoms and signs noted by the advanced practice nursing practitioner not only in the context of his chronic pain and the meaning of that pain but also as expressions of Jamie's unique individuality.

The advanced practice nursing practitioner made a decision by reasoning each element of the pain history schema map over and over in her mind, and observing Jamie's demeanour that a high tech pain infusion was not a priority at this time, even though Jamie verbalised his disappointment profusely. Does the reasoned decision by the advanced practice nursing practitioner seem out of sync with the third dimension of person-centered care, 'sharing power and responsibility'? Jamie was asked to voice his thoughts, that were listened to intently and his involvement was encouraged, but genuinely my advanced nursing skills and knowledge predominated, reflected also in a reasoned decision to seek a cardiology opinion. The clinical encounter is a paradigm of ethics-based relationships, which builds on awareness of the other *qua* other, and is concerned with fulfilling the therapeutic mandate (Kottow 2001, p. 53). Caring for the other means doing one's best to help her/him, so that care and cure are inextricably interwoven, although care is the more fundamental form of human relatedness (Kottow 2001, p. 53). According to Mead and Bower (2000) 'it is unclear to what degree the clinician-patient relationship can in practice become genuinely symmetrical, as patient-centered care is concerned to encourage significantly greater patient involvement in care than is generally associated with the biomedical model' (p. 1090). A referral to an advanced practice nursing practitioner in cardiology was processed, who agreed to review Jamie immediately. Approximately, 40 minutes later, Jamie returned to the pain department and informed the advanced practice nursing practitioner (pain medicine) he was scheduled for an angiogram later that day as there was 'something but nothing specific on the ECG'. The advanced practice nursing practitioner (cardiology) later confirmed that some non-specific changes were evident on the ECG and the angiogram was the recommended evidence-based approach in this instance.

In my role as the advanced practice nursing practitioner I contacted the primary care physician by telephone, who listened attentively and suggested that the history did not fit the classification of cardiac pain in this case. Based on this conversation, I reflected on the entire episode, I did not question my judgement or decision, except to state that I would await the outcome of the angiogram and learn from the process, think about how it could be managed differently, and modify my actions in the-here-and-now if relevant. In my world of clinical practice, the patient is front and centre in all situations. I was the lead practitioner of Jamie's care at that point. I also had an intrinsic understanding of the illness experience in the here-and-now and the uniqueness of the narrative expressed by Jamie in his pain diary:

> *I am experiencing chronic neck and shoulder pain. This pain seems to emanate from the base of my skull (right hand side) and move downwards through the thoracic spine and outwards through the sternum and the rib cage. It is brought on by activity that I can barely walk. On a pain scale 1-10; I am talking about 20. None of the treatment has eased this pain, same pain for the past few months. I have been investigated upside down and nothing new comes or emerges except my bank balance seems to become depleted.*

I get 2-3 days relief from the infusions, and then back to the same. All this pain persists despite the fact that I am on strong painkillers. Nobody has been able to pinpoint the root of the problem. This in my opinion is due to the fact that nobody is really listening to me. Each person has his/her own theory and they all differ. There is no joined up thinking. All the medical opinion says my pains, neck, shoulder, chest, arm is unconnected but I assure you they are connected in some way.

As it stands I have no quality of life. I go from painkiller to painkiller, from injection to injection, from drip to drip. I am unable to do my work; I regularly go home because the pain is so severe. My home life and that of my family suffers greatly. I feel abandoned.

By definition, pain is subjective and a highly personal experience, which presented a challenge in its measurement for me, thereby relying on Jamie's self-report and his demeanour to provide a glimpse of this somewhat atypical pain presentation. Therefore, many theories from psychology, pain medicine, and experimental research were confronted and transformed from various disciplines to inform Jamie's pain care. However, in the borrowing and application of this knowledge, the advanced practice nursing practitioner assembled the patient portrait, integrating different perspectives holistically, inclusive of Jamie's written and verbal narrative. The fourth dimension in the person-centered framework is 'the therapeutic alliance' (Mead and Bower 2000). In this case, it would seem that the therapeutic alliance has shifted as Jamie acknowledged positively and emotionally that the pending angiogram may indirectly improve his condition and reduce his 'current suffering'. Hobbs (2009) postulates that within a patient-centered encounter, therapeutic engagement is a cyclical process based on the development of trust. When the process of therapeutic engagement is successful, the patient receives effective care that lessens suffering and ensures that their needs are met (Hobbs 2009, p. 57). It is no surprise according to Hobbs (2009) that therapeutic engagement is composed of knowing the patient and developing a relationship (p. 58). Central to the clinical judgement of expert nurses is what they describe in their everyday discourse as knowing the patient, i.e. knowing the patient's typical pattern of responses and knowing the patient as a person (Benner et al. 1996; Tanner et al. 1993; Thomas and Fothergill-Bourbonnais 2005). This experientially gained clinical knowledge sensitises the nurse to potential issues and concerns in particular situations (Benner et al. 1996; Benner 1984). Using this particularistic knowledge of the patient, nurses formulate a sequence of clinical judgements about the patient's status and potential, upon which they base their choice of intervention strategies (O'Connor 2012; Jenny and Logan 1992). Furthermore, knowing the patient is equated with nursing 'gestalt' which was found by Pyles and Stern (1983) to be a process used by experienced critical care nurses whereby fundamental knowledge, past experiences, cue identification and sensory clues were linked, leading to a categorisation of the patient picture that involved a synergy of logic and intuition. However, part of the complexity of clinical judgement and decision-making in this exemplar case is the atypical chest pain presentation alongside trying to unpack an acute pain event from chronic pain and no pain epicentre identified by Jamie pertinent to the pain experience. Therefore, the atypical pain pattern was compared to the atypical pain self-reports from previous pain episodes integrated with the history and physical exam, so something unique was implicit that convinced the advanced practice nursing practitioner in the absence of concrete signs, that something was amiss. That said, Jamie's frustration was also unusual when the advanced practice nursing practitioner was concentrating to forensically unravel the pain history, an atypical behaviour that was also conceived as a 'qualifying factor' in her knowledge of the patient and building a picture portrait mosaic to ascertain a pain diagnosis.

Patients are assumed to have a "compromised physiological state" and a "threatened identity" because they often experience a lack of control and/or feel alienated (Hobbs 2009, p. 55). Consequently, nurses need to reduce suffering and alleviate vulnerabilities through a process of caring in the clinical encounter. Hudon et al. (2012) emphasised the importance of legitimising the patient's experience of chronic illness, which means nurses invite patients to express their doubts, concerns, and feelings of loss and grief and suffering. This is the approach that the advanced practice nursing practitioner assumed throughout the clinical encounter with Jamie. When the struggles with their illness are acknowledged, patients are assumed to feel "relieved" (Hudon et al. 2012, p. 173). Of note, the advanced practice nursing practitioner was privileged to be able to acknowledge Jamie's expression of pain and its associated impact on his day-to day activities or lack of by reading and re-reading the pain diary that informed the essence of his current care trajectory.

In this instance the advanced practice nursing practitioner and the patient shared a history and as a result Jamie felt known as an individual. This dimension of patient-centered care is communication; knowing the patient, and acknowledgement that all members of a team affect the team's relationship with the patient. Effective communication must begin with active listening—emphatically attuning to both the patient's medical and non-medical needs (e.g., values, fears, life events)—that can have a major impact on both the process and outcomes of the interaction (Greene et al. 2012, p. 52).

A case study-based observational interaction analysis of verbal communication and verbal social interactions, arising from 30 primary health care nurse practitioner consultations was undertaken by Barratt and Thomas (2018) to determine the discrete nature of social interactions occurring in nurse practitioner consultations and investigate the relationship between consultation social interaction styles (biomedical and patient-centered). The findings demonstrate that in the opening phase no significant differences in the frequency of usage of patient-centered style interactions amongst nurse practitioners and patients were observed. In the history phase nurse practitioners were significantly more likely to use patient-centered style interactions than patients. In the exam phase nurse practitioners were significantly more likely to use biomedical style interactions than the patients (Barratt and Thomas 2018). In the counsel phase of the consultations the patients used significantly more patient-centered style interactions than the nurse practitioners, such as showing agreement or giving psychosocial information. In the counsel phase of the consultations nurse practitioners were significantly more likely to use biomedical style interactions than the patients, such as counselling regarding therapeutics and checking for understanding. In the study, nurse practitioners and patients were both found to have no significant differences in their overall respective usage of patient-centered interactions (Barratt and Thomas 2018). Furthermore, a larger proportion (66.7%) of the consultations were conducted in a congruent interaction style, meaning that both patients and nurse practitioners synchronically used the same style of interactions, with the majority of those congruent consultations comprising patient-centered style interactions (Barratt and Thomas 2018).

Subsequent to the angiogram, Jamie was scheduled for an angioplasty and stenting; five stents were placed within 24 hours of this clinical encounter in the department of pain medicine; one stent to the right coronary artery, three stents to left anterior descending artery and a further stent in the left circumflex. The knowledge of this outcome provoked the advanced practice nursing practitioner to deliberate on the following question; 'What if I had given Jamie the high-tech pain infusion … and a cardiac event ensued in the hospital surroundings. … where does the concept accountable sit'? The point to be made here is that 'What If?' does not provoke emancipatory learning for an advanced practice nursing practitioner, it just constricts any learning that might ensue in such a paradigm case. The key issue here was the generation of personal knowledge and the sharing of this with the primary care physician and colleagues at a subsequent interdisciplinary case conference. The attention of the advanced practice nursing practitioner was not to ask of her and colleagues what worked and did not work. The attention was focused on specific evidence-based solutions in pain practice associated with the case and self-reflection on the learning process rather than only on the outcome. When this skilful reflective process is also self-monitored and self-evaluated, it is called self-regulated learning (Kreber 2002).

The primary care physician was knowledgeable regarding Jamie and was very conversant with his medical history spanning over 10 years. This case is not an example of dominance and or substitution of an advanced practice nursing practitioner's judgement and that of the primary care physician or in fact, drawing any comparisons between both professionals and professions. The paradigm case illustrates a much more subtle and interprofessional collaborative partnership between professionals at an advanced level of practice and scope of practice, utilising a higher order of capability in the complex landscape of clinical practice. The conversation with the primary care physician enabled the advanced practice nursing practitioner defend her care, clinical reasoning, clinical judgement and evidence-based decision-making based on here-and-now thinking through use of the patient history, physical exam, relevant theories and the diary narrative that informed her judgement. The final dimension in the person-centered care framework is referred to as 'nurse-as-person'. According to Mead and Bower (2000) 'doctor-as-person' concerns the influence of the personal qualities of the doctor. In this exemplar case the advanced practice nursing practitioner proposes that the indicators associated with critical reflectivity were her enablers aligned with personal qualities such as; honesty, integrity, courage, open-mindedness, perseverance, and humility and an ethical stance of 'compassion' to understand as the case unfolded, and ultimately to care for Jamie safely and expertly. Compassion according to Pellegrino and Thomasma (1993) "focuses on co-experiencing another's suffering; it includes an ability to objectify what another person is feeling in symbolic form, that is, in our speech, our body language and in our participation in the 'story' of the other's illness" (p. 82).

To embed this exemplar case in the context of advanced nursing practice, I, as the clinical professor/advanced practice nursing practitioner argue is about fostering the 'perceiving eye' in the patient encounter. A central feature of the care philosophy of Martinsen (2006) is her emphasis on perception in our interaction with others, as well as in clinical situations, and considers perception to constitute an important part of clinical judgement, where we are touched and emotionally involved before we understand the needs of the other. Further, Martinsen explores different dimensions of the clinical gaze and draws a distinction between perceiving and recording (Martinsen 2006). The recording eye is reductionist and neutral such as categorising physiological cues, whereas the perceiving eye opens for "a seeing emotion". Therefore, the dominant gaze during the history and physical exam conducted by the advanced practice nursing practitioner was with the 'recording eye'. The 'recording eye' is powerful during the process of obtaining facts to reach a diagnosis which is very important in this paradigm case. On the other hand, the 'perceiving eye' according to Martinsen (2006) can strengthen the patient's life courage and in that instance the person will feel they were heard and do not feel abandoned in the clinical encounter. I am reminded of Jamie's narrative in the pain diary and his demeanour throughout the clinical episode of care. Moreover, the fostering of the 'perceiving eye' may facilitate care in each clinical encounter, may further contribute to protecting the integrity of patients, as well as refining clinical proficiency (Martinsen 2011). In this clinical encounter with Jamie, the advanced practice nursing practitioner utilised the lens of the 'recording gaze' and the 'lens of the perceiving gaze'. The lens of the 'perceiving gaze' moved the advanced practice nursing practitioner to something in the patient's demeanour and in being aware of her own 'seeing emotions' in meeting with Jamie, she captured important information regarding the essence of the clinical situation. This awareness motivated the advanced practice nursing practitioner to defer the high-tech pain infusion and initiate a further cardiology work-up. The particular theories used throughout this case by the advanced practice nursing practitioner; informal, personal, experiential, and formal were constructed and transformed based on reflection-in-action and reflection-on-action and the need to seek answers to inform her advanced reasoning, judgement and decision-making and to keep Jamie safe and secure throughout the clinical encounter and on transition to home. According to Rolfe (1997) theory and practice are one, and the reflexive practitioner is both researcher and theory-builder (p. 97). Further, an understanding of the many factors such as demographic, genetic, psychosocial and biological that produces a mosaic that uniquely contributes to pain in each individual patient is critical for effective pain assessment and pain management. This understanding serves as a foundation for personalised pain treatment and as yet an unrealised goal (Fillingham 2017).

More importantly, the very nature of nursing practice necessitates hearing and understanding the language of others, especially the language of meaning that patients assign to their experience. Scholarship requires making that understanding conscious (Diers 1995, p. 25), an important remit for all advanced practice nursing practitioners/aspirants.

7.3   Conclusion

The exemplar case analysed by a joint-chair of clinical nursing advanced practice nursing practitioner is explored. The complex case tested the registered advanced practice nursing practitioner and prescriber on several levels, and equally it could be interpreted that the patient was also tested in the context of their chronic pain trajectory. A patient-centered five-dimensional framework was adapted; 'biopsy-chosocial perspective', 'the patient-as-person', 'sharing power and responsibility', 'the therapeutic alliance', and 'the nurse-as-person' (Mead and Bower 2000).

The subtleties of the case as it unfolded and the complexity of interpreting the covert and overt cues are mirrored throughout the advanced clinical reasoning, judgement and decision making employed by the advanced practice nursing practitioner. Reflection-in-action and on-action is kernel to the case, while acknowledging the patient as an active participant that necessitated the utilisation of a schema of informal, formal and experiential theories on the part of the advanced practice nursing practitioner.

Finally, engagement in clinical practice by a professor with a PhD, who is an advanced practice nursing practitioner with prescriptive authority is a worthy platform for Boyer's dimensions of scholarship; discovery, integration, teaching, application, and engagement and an appropriate action agenda for 'what matters most to the patient as an individual' is 'what matters most to the nurse' in partnership with disciplines who have a similar patient-centered evidence-based action agenda. Of note, the nature of scholarship, a career legacy map and advanced practice are an important triad to nurture and sustain a person-centered culture' in challenging, unpredictable, and sometimes vulnerable but precious moments in the health care setting of the patient/client and in the complex clinical milieu of the advanced practice nursing practitioner/aspirant.

References

Barratt J, Thomas N. Nurse practitioner consultations in primary health care: an observational interaction analysis of social interactions and consultation outcomes. Prim Health Care Res Dev. 2018;6:1. https://doi.org/10.1017/S1463423618000427. https://www.cambridge.org/phc.

Benner P. From novice to expert: excellence and power in clinical nursing practice. Menlo-Park, CA: Addison-Wesley; 1984.

Benner P, Tanner C, Chesla C. Expertise in nursing practice: caring, clinical judgement and ethics. New York, NY: Springer Publishing Company; 1996.

Bond M, Breivik H, Jensen TS, Scholten W, Soyannwo O, Treede RD. Pain associated with neurological disorders. In: Aarli JA, Dua T, Janca A, Muscetta A, editors. Neurological disorders: public health challenges. Geneva: WHO Press; 2006. p. 127–39.

Bonica J. The management of pain. Philadelphia, PA: Lea & Febiger; 1953.

Breivik H, Collett B, Ventafridda V, Cohen R, Gallacher D. Survey of chronic pain in Europe: prevalence, impact on daily life, and treatment. Eur J Pain. 2006;10:87.

Darbyshire P. Joint or clinical chairs in nursing: from cup of plenty to poisoned chalice? J Adv Nurs. 2010;66:2592–9.

Diers D. Clinical scholarship. J Prof Nurs. 1995;11:24–30.

Dominick C, Blyth F, Nicholas M. Unpacking the burden: understanding the relationships between chronic pain and comorbidity in the general population. Pain. 2012;153:293–304.

Fillingham R. Individual differences in pain: understanding the mosaic that makes pain personal. Pain. 2017;158:S11–8.

Gatchel R, Peng Y, Peters M, Fuchs P, Turk D. The biopsychosocial approach to chronic pain: scientific advances and future directions. Psychol Bull. 2007;133:581–624.

Goldberg D, Summer J. Pain as a global public health priority. BMC Public Health. 2011;11:770.

Gore M, Sadosky A, Stacey B, Tai K, Leslie D. The burden of chronic low back pain: clinical comorbidities, treatment patterns, and health care costs in usual care settings. Spine. 2012;37:e668–77.

Greene S, Tuzzio L, Cherkin D. A framework for making patient-centered care front and center. Perm J. 2012;16:49–53.

Gureje O, Von Korff M, Kola L, Demyttenaere K, He Y, Posada-Villa J, Lepine JP, Angermeyer MC, Levinson D, de Girolamo G, Iwata N, Karam A, Guimaraes Borges GL, de Graaf R, Browne MO, Stein DJ, Haro JM, Bromet EJ, Kessler RC, Alonso J. The relation between multiple pains and mental disorders: results from the World Mental Health Surveys. Pain. 2008;135:82–91.

Hobbs J. A dimensional analysis of patient-centered care. Nurs Res. 2009;58:52–62.

Hudon C, Fortin M, Haggerty J, Loignon C, Lambert M, Poitras M. Patient-centered care in chronic disease management: a thematic analysis of the literature in family medicine. Patient Educ Couns. 2012;88:170–6.

Illingworth R. What does patient-centered mean in relation to the consultation? Clin Teach. 2010;7:116–20.

Institute of Medicine (IOM). Relieving pain in America: a blueprint for transforming prevention, care, education, and research. Washington, DC: The National Academies Press; 2011.

Jenny J, Logan J. Knowing the patient: one aspect of clinical knowledge. Image. 1992;24:254–8.

Kirsh K. Differentiating and managing common psychiatric comorbidities seen in chronic pain patients. J Pain Palliat Care Pharmacother. 2010;24:39–47.

Kottow M. Between curing and caring. Nurs Philos. 2001;2:53–61.

Kreber C. Teaching excellence, teaching expertise, and the scholarship of teaching. Innov High Educ. 2002;27:5–23.

Martinsen K. Care and vulnerability. Oslo: Akribe; 2006.

Martinsen E. Care for nurses only: medicine and the perceiving eye. Health Care Annal. 2011;19:115–27.

Mead N, Bower P. Patient-centeredness: a conceptual framework and review of the empirical literature. Soc Sci Med. 2000;31:1087–110.

Merskey H, Bogduk N. Classification of chronic pain: descriptions of chronic pain syndromes and definitions of pain terms. Washington, DC: International Association for the Study of Pain, IASP; 1994.

Nicholas M, Vlaeyen J, Pliel W, Barke A, Aziz Q, Bienoliel R, Cohen M, et al. The IASP classification of chronic pain for ICD-11: chronic primary pain. Pain. 2019;160:28–37.

O'Connor L. Critical care nurses' judgement of pain status: a case study design. Intensive Crit Care Nurs. 2012;28:215–23.

Page M, Fortier M, Ware M, Choiniere M. As if one pain problem was not enough: prevalence and patterns of co-existing chronic pain conditions and their impact on treatment outcomes. J Pain Res. 2018;11:237–54.

Pellegrino E, Thomasma D. Virtues in medical practice. New York, NY: Oxford University Press; 1993.

Pizzo P, Clarke N. Alleviating suffering 101-pain relief in United States. N Engl J Med. 2012;366:197–9.

Pyles S, Stern P. Discovery of nursing gestalt in critical care nursing: the importance of the gray gorilla syndrome. Image. 1983;XV:51–7.

Rolfe G. Beyond expertise: theory, practice and the reflexive practitioner. J Clin Nurs. 1997;6:93–7.

Schon D. The reflective practitioner. London: Temple Smith; 1983.

Schopflocker D, Taenzer P, Jovey R. The prevalence of chronic pain in Canada. Pain Res Manag. 2011;16:445–50.

Tanenbaum S. What is patient-centered care? A typology of models and missions. Health Care Anal. 2013;23:272–87.

Tanner C, Benner P, Chesla C, Gordon D. The phenomenology of knowing the patient. Image. 1993;25:273–80.

Thomas M, Fothergill-Bourbonnais F. Clinical judgements about endotracheal suctioning: what cues do expert paediatric critical care nurses consider? Crit Care Nurs Clin North Am. 2005;17:329–40.

Treede R, Pliel W, Barke A, Aziz Q, Bennett M, Benioliel R, Cohen M, Evers S, et al. A classification of chronic pain. Pain. 2015;156:1003–7.

Van Hecke O, Torrance N, Smith B. Chronic pain epidemiology and its clinical relevance. Br J Anaseth. 2013;111:13–8.